Stephan E.R. Domayer

Monitoring of Cartilage Repair in the Knee

Stephan E.R. Domayer

Monitoring of Cartilage Repair in the Knee

In vivo T2 mapping and dGEMRIC at 3.0 Tesla

Südwestdeutscher Verlag für Hochschulschriften

Impressum/Imprint (nur für Deutschland/only for Germany)
Bibliografische Information der Deutschen Nationalbibliothek: Die Deutsche Nationalbibliothek verzeichnet diese Publikation in der Deutschen Nationalbibliografie; detaillierte bibliografische Daten sind im Internet über http://dnb.d-nb.de abrufbar.
Alle in diesem Buch genannten Marken und Produktnamen unterliegen warenzeichen-, marken- oder patentrechtlichem Schutz bzw. sind Warenzeichen oder eingetragene Warenzeichen der jeweiligen Inhaber. Die Wiedergabe von Marken, Produktnamen, Gebrauchsnamen, Handelsnamen, Warenbezeichnungen u.s.w. in diesem Werk berechtigt auch ohne besondere Kennzeichnung nicht zu der Annahme, dass solche Namen im Sinne der Warenzeichen- und Markenschutzgesetzgebung als frei zu betrachten wären und daher von jedermann benutzt werden dürften.

Coverbild: www.ingimage.com

Verlag: Südwestdeutscher Verlag für Hochschulschriften GmbH & Co. KG
Dudweiler Landstr. 99, 66123 Saarbrücken, Deutschland
Telefon +49 681 37 20 271-1, Telefax +49 681 37 20 271-0
Email: info@svh-verlag.de

Approved by: Wien, MUW, Diss., 2011

Herstellung in Deutschland:
Schaltungsdienst Lange o.H.G., Berlin
Books on Demand GmbH, Norderstedt
Reha GmbH, Saarbrücken
Amazon Distribution GmbH, Leipzig
ISBN: 978-3-8381-2896-2

Imprint (only for USA, GB)
Bibliographic information published by the Deutsche Nationalbibliothek: The Deutsche Nationalbibliothek lists this publication in the Deutsche Nationalbibliografie; detailed bibliographic data are available in the Internet at http://dnb.d-nb.de.
Any brand names and product names mentioned in this book are subject to trademark, brand or patent protection and are trademarks or registered trademarks of their respective holders. The use of brand names, product names, common names, trade names, product descriptions etc. even without a particular marking in this works is in no way to be construed to mean that such names may be regarded as unrestricted in respect of trademark and brand protection legislation and could thus be used by anyone.

Cover image: www.ingimage.com

Publisher: Südwestdeutscher Verlag für Hochschulschriften GmbH & Co. KG
Dudweiler Landstr. 99, 66123 Saarbrücken, Germany
Phone +49 681 37 20 271-1, Fax +49 681 37 20 271-0
Email: info@svh-verlag.de

Printed in the U.S.A.
Printed in the U.K. by (see last page)
ISBN: 978-3-8381-2896-2

Copyright © 2011 by the author and Südwestdeutscher Verlag für Hochschulschriften GmbH & Co. KG and licensors
All rights reserved. Saarbrücken 2011

Acknowledgments

Research relies on the interdisciplinary contribution of all the people who participate in it. I have been very lucky to work in a field with several experts with complementary skills who were willing to teach me.
Professor Stefan Nehrer, M.D. and PD Ronald Dorotka, M.D. introduced me to the field of cartilage repair research; it is due to their skilled teaching that I learned to organize clinical studies. I owe them a debt of gratitude for the knowledge that lead me to combine MRI and clinical cartilage repair research at Medical University of Vienna.
After my M.D. program was completed, Professor Siegfried Trattnig, M.D. agreed to collaborate with the Department of Orthopedics at Medical University of Vienna. He gave me the opportunity to start the PhD program under his supervision. He has been a diligent mentor ever since; encouraging and open to new ideas but always ready to accurately evaluate and correct my work. I have learned to know and to appreciate his communication skills, his generosity to share his knowledge and his expertise in the formation and handling of research groups. His enthusiasm and skills in research will always be an example to follow.
Research on the studies included in this thesis had just started when Professor Rainer Kotz, M.D. gave me the chance to enter the residency program in October 2006. It had always been my goal to learn the skills of orthopedic surgery at his department, and since then a never ending wealth of clinical knowledge, experiences and skills have been offered to me. I was always given the time and flexibility to pursue the PhD program and clinical research during the residency. It is because of Professor Kotz I was able to not only receive outstanding training as orthopedic surgeon, but complete my PhD as well. I would like to thank Professor Kotz for his support in this endeavor. His skills and knowledge will always be a measure for my clinical work.
Though my decision to study medicine was never in doubt, I had a great interest in physics as well. The PhD program offered me to get a basic understanding of the complex and extensive field of medical physics, but more importantly, it offered me a chance to work closely with those who are highly regarded in this field. I would like to particularly thank Professor Ewald Moser, PhD for the chance to participate in the PhD medical physics program and for his continuing support. His precise assessment of scientific parameters and his constant readiness to rethink established concepts has been inspirational.
There are numerous other people who contributed to my training and research. Among them I would like to thank, in alphabetic order, Klaus Friedrich, M.D., Clemens Hirschfeld, M.D., Vladimir Juras, Ph.D., Florian Kutscha-Lissberg, M.D., Charles Mamisch, M.D., Catherine Matero, David Stelzeneder M.D., Pavol Szomolanyi, PhD and Götz Welsch, M.D. .
Above all, clinical medical science requires a wealth of support at home. My stunning and beloved wife Carina, who agreed to sacrifice numerous weekends in support of this thesis, encouraged and inspired me to keep at. I thank her for the last five years and for her incredible generosity and patience.

Stephan Domayer, M.D.

Disclosure

There was no conflict of interest with regard to affiliations with any organization or entity that had interest in the outcome of the respective studies. None of the authors were affiliated with stock ownership, employment or honoraria except Professor Avner Yayon, ProChon Biotech Ltd. who participated in writing the methods section of the manuscript 'T2 mapping and dGEMRIC of reparative cartilage after autologous chondrocyte implantation with a fibrin based scaffold in the knee: preliminary results'. Project funding was mainly covered by the pre-existent infrastructure of the involved departments of the Medical University of Vienna. Additional funding was received by the FWF Austrian Science Fund, project numbers FWF-TRP-Project L243-B15 and FWF P 18110-B1.

This thesis consists both of data from several published studies that were conducted by the candidate or that he contributed to; furthermore, unpublished data sets have been implemented to prove methodological aspects and to augment the correlation analyses. Novel knowledge therefore derives from the cumulative evaluation of source data.

The introduction first treats the background from the view of orthopedic clinical research on cartilage repair and then gives a short overview of the relevant MRI technology. The Results Sections are organized in adherence to the original publication data. Subsequently the interpretation of the results, possible implications for clinical research in the field of orthopaedic surgery but also potential pitfalls and intrinsic shortcomings ot the MRI techniques are discussed.

The publications that were included (in chronologic order):

1: Trattnig S, Domayer S, Welsch GW, Mosher T, Eckstein F.
MR imaging of cartilage and its repair in the knee - a review.
Eur Radiol. 2009 Mar 13.

2: Domayer SE, Welsch GH, Nehrer S, Chiari C, Dorotka R, Szomolanyi P, Mamisch TC, Yayon A, Trattnig S.
T2 mapping and dGEMRIC after autologous chondrocyte implantation with a fibrin-based scaffold in the knee: Preliminary results.
Eur J Radiol. 2009 Jan 19.

3: Domayer SE, Welsch GH, Dorotka R, Mamisch TC, Marlovits S, Szomolanyi P, Trattnig S.
MRI monitoring of cartilage repair in the knee: a review.
Semin Musculoskelet Radiol. 2008 Dec;12(4):302-17.

4: Domayer SE, Kutscha-Lissberg F, Welsch G, Dorotka R, Nehrer S, Gäbler C, Mamisch TC, Trattnig S.
T2 mapping in the knee after microfracture at 3.0 T: correlation of global T2 values and clinical outcome - preliminary results.
Osteoarthritis Cartilage. 2008 Aug;16(8):903-8.

5: Trattnig S, Mamisch TC, Pinker K, Domayer S, Szomolanyi P, Marlovits S, Kutscha-Lissberg F, Welsch GH.
Differentiating normal hyaline cartilage from post-surgical repair tissue using fast gradient echo imaging in delayed gadolinium-enhanced MRI (dGEMRIC) at 3 Tesla.
Eur Radiol. 2008 Jun;18(6):1251-9.

6: Welsch GH, Mamisch TC, Domayer SE, Dorotka R, Kutscha-Lissberg F, Marlovits S, White LM, Trattnig S.
Cartilage T2 assessment at 3-T MR imaging: in vivo differentiation of normal

hyaline cartilage from reparative tissue after two cartilage repair procedures--initial experience.
Radiology. 2008 Apr;247(1):154-61.

All authors consented to the inclusion and further evaluation of the published data as found in the thesis. In the sections that concern published data, the reference is given in the beginning; all unpublished data have been collected, evaluated and interpreted by the candidate.

Stephan Domayer, M.D.

Abbreviations

ACI	Autologous Chondrocyte Implantation
BMI	Body Mass Index
CA	Contrast Agent
dGEMRIC	delayed Gadolinium enhanced MRI of cartilage
FOV	Field of View
GAG	Glycosaminoglycan
MACT	Matrix associated Autologous Chondrocyte Transplantation
MESE	Multi-Echo Spin-Echo
MFX	Microfracture
MRI	Magnetic Resonance Imaging
R1	Relaxation Rate
ΔR1	Delta relaxation Rate
rΔR1	Relative Delta Relaxation Rate
ROI	Region of Interest
RC	Reference Cartilage
RT	Repair Tissue
rT2	Relative T2
TE	Echo Time
TR	Repetition Time

Contents

1 ABSTRACTS 5

1.1 ENGLISH 5
1.1.1 BACKGROUND 5
1.1.2 MATERIAL AND METHODS 5
1.1.3 RESULTS 5
1.1.4 DISCUSSION 6

1.2 GERMAN 7
1.2.1 HINTERGRUND 7
1.2.2 MATERIAL UND METHODEN 7
1.2.3 ERGEBNISSE 7
1.2.4 DISKUSSION 8

2 INTRODUCTION 9

2.1 BASIC CARTILAGE BIOLOGY 9
2.2 CARTILAGE DEFECTS IN THE KNEE 9
2.3 SURGICAL CARTILAGE REPAIR 10
2.3.1 MOSAICPLASTY 11
2.3.2 MICROFRACTURE 12
2.3.3 ACI AND MACT 12
2.3.4 CARTILAGE REPAIR – COMPARISON OF SURGICAL TECHNIQUES 13
2.3.5 REPAIR TISSUE COMPOSITION AND CONSEQUENCES FOR CLINICAL APPLICATION 15
2.3.6 REPAIR TISSUE BIOPSY – ASPECTS FOR CLINICAL RESEARCH 17

2.4 MRI OF CARTILAGE 17
2.4.1 MORPHOLOGIC MRI 17
2.4.2 MR MAPPING 19

2.5 MRI IN CARTILAGE REPAIR 25
2.5.1 MORPHOLOGIC MRI 25
2.5.2 MORPHOLOGIC MRI ASSESSMENT OF MICROFRACTURE, MOSAICPLASTY AND ACI [89] 25
2.5.3 MORPHOLOGIC RATING 32

2.5.4   T2 MAPPING – DEVELOPMENT IN CLINICAL USE 33
2.5.5   T2 MAPPING – FIRST APPLICATIONS IN CARTILAGE REPAIR 33
2.5.6   T2 MAPPING – METHODOLOGICAL STUDIES 35
2.5.7   DGEMRIC – CLINICAL USE 37
2.5.8   DGEMRIC FOR THE ASSESSMENT OF CARTILAGE REPAIR 37
2.5.9   DGEMRIC – METHODOLOGICAL STUDIES 38
2.6   MR SAFETY 41
2.7   CONCLUSION 42

3   HYPOTHESES 44

3.1   DESIGN 45
3.2   LIMITATIONS 45

4   METHODS 46

4.1   PATIENT RECRUITMENT 46
4.2   CARTILAGE SURGERY 46
4.2.1   MICROFRACTURE 46
4.2.2   MACT: HYALOGRAFT C 47
4.2.3   MACT: BIOCART II 48
4.2.4   REHABILITATION 49
4.3   MRI 50
4.3.1   MRI UNIT SPECIFICATIONS 50
4.3.2   MEASUREMENT METHODS AND SAFETY CONSIDERATIONS 50
4.3.3   MORPHOLOGIC ASSESSMENT 51
4.3.4   DGEMRIC 51
4.3.5   T2 MAPPING 53
4.4   CLINICAL EVALUATION 55
4.4.1   LYSHOLM KNEE SCORE 55
4.4.2   IKDC RATING 55
4.5   ETHICAL CONSIDERATIONS 56
4.6   FUNDING AND CONFLICT OF INTEREST 56
4.7   STATISTICAL EVALUATION 57
4.8   STUDY PLAN 58

4.8.1 SEQUENCE VALIDATION 58
4.8.2 CASE SERIES TO EVALUATE FEASIBILITY AND RANGE OF EFFECT SIZES 58
4.8.3 CORRELATION ANALYSES OF CLINICAL OUTCOME AND MRI EFFECT SIZES 59

5 RESULTS 60

5.1 SEQUENCE VALIDATION STUDIES 60
5.1.1 T1 - VIBE SEQUENCE 60
5.1.2 T2 MULTI ECHO SPIN ECHO VALIDATION 65
5.2 FEASIBILITY IN VIVO – OBSERVATIONAL CASE SERIES STUDIES 67
5.2.1 OVERVIEW OF THE CLINICAL CASES 67
5.2.2 HYALOGRAFT C - 10 CASES 69
5.2.3 T2 MAPPING AND DGEMRIC OF REPARATIVE CARTILAGE AFTER AUTOLOGOUS CHONDROCYTE IMPLANTATION WITH A FIBRIN BASED SCAFFOLD IN THE KNEE: PRELIMINARY RESULTS [160] 70
5.2.4 CROSS-SECTIONAL CASES SERIES COMPARING MICROFRACTURE AND HYALOGRAFT REPAIR TISSUE T2 PROPERTIES [161] 72
5.2.5 DIFFERENTIATING NORMAL HYALINE CARTILAGE FROM POST-SURGICAL REPAIR TISSUE USING FAST GRADIENT ECHO IMAGING IN DELAYED GADOLINIUM-ENHANCED MRI (DGEMRIC) AT 3 T [162] 74
5.3 CORRELATION OF T1 AND T2 WITH CLINICAL OUTCOME 75
5.3.1 METHODS 75
5.3.2 T1 – CUMULATIVE EVALUATION 76
5.3.3 T2 – CUMULATIVE EVALUATION 77
5.4 CARTILAGE REPAIR TISSUE QUALITY ASSESSMENT WITH T2 MAPPING 79

6 DISCUSSION 80

6.1 OVERVIEW 80
6.2 METHODOLOGICAL CONSIDERATIONS 81
6.3 CASE SERIES: CLINICS AND MRI 86
6.3.1 THE CASE SERIES IN THE CONTEXT OF CLINICAL CARTILAGE REPAIR RESEARCH 86
6.4 CORRELATION OF T1 AND T2 WITH CLINICAL OUTCOME 90
6.4.1 T1 90
6.4.2 T2 91

6.5   CONSIDERATIONS ON THE USE OF DGEMRIC AND OF T2 MAPPING IN CLINICAL
RESEARCH AND ROUTINE 94
6.6   LIMITATIONS AND LEVEL OF EVIDENCE 97
6.7   OUTLOOK 98
6.8   CONCLUSION 99

7   TABLES 101

8   FIGURES 104

9   REFERENCES 122

1 Abstracts

1.1 English

1.1.1 Background

A variety of surgical options to treat cartilage defects are currently available, however data on the efficacy remain sparse. Recent progress in MRI technology has yielded techniques designed to directly visualize the molecular ultrastructure of cartilage. Such technology could be used to assess cartilage repair tissue and provide a new evaluation tool for clinical cartilage repair research.

1.1.2 Material and Methods

After the successful validation of a new T1 mapping sequence for delayed Gadolinium Enhanced MRI of Cartilage (dGEMRIC) in phantoms, T2-mapping and dGEMRIC were used at 3.0 Tesla (3T) to perform several pilot studies in patients after various cartilage repair surgery techniques of the knee for the first time. Clinical scores and parameters were assessed at the time of MR exams in order to estimate effect sizes in clinical research aside the validation of the sequences.

1.1.3 Results

Both dGEMRIC and T2-mapping could differentiate between native cartilage and repair tissue as well as between repair tissue after a variety of cartilage surgery techniques. However, T1 and T2 are subject to a highly individual variability, which indicates that native cartilage and repair tissue within the joint must be compared in order to attain coherent data. Relative T2 correlates with clinical outcome, whereas T1 does not, in the course of cross sectional studies.

1.1.4 Discussion

Both T2 mapping and dGEMRIC are objective, reproducible and above all non-invasive techniques to assess cartilage repair tissue ultrastructure that can be used to differentiate between multiple surgical techniques. Despite a number of possible error sources, MR mapping can provide an additional effect size for the evaluation of cartilage repair surgery efficacy. Preliminary data assessed in the course of this thesis indicate that quantitative MRI parameters can improve the efficacy of clinical research.

1.2 German

1.2.1 Hintergrund

Derzeit ist eine Reihe chirurgischer Optionen zur Behandlung von Knorpeldefekten verfügbar; die Datenlage über die Effizenz bleibt jedoch unzufriedenstellend. Neu entwickelte MR Techniken ermöglichen die direkte Visualisierung der molekularen Ultrastruktur von Gelenksknorpel. Damit könnte Knorpelreparaturgewebe objektiv und non-invasiv evaluiert werden und die geeigneten MR Techniken als Evaluationsinstrument in der klinischen Knorpelforschung dienen.

1.2.2 Material und Methoden

Nach Validierung einer neuen T1-mapping Sequenz für ´delayed Gadolinium Enhanced MRI of Cartilage´ (dGEMRIC) in Phantomstudien wurden T2 mapping und dGEMRIC erstmals bei 3.0 Tesla für mehrere Pilotstudien am Patienten nach verschiedenen knorpelchirurgischen Verfahren im Knie verwendet. Klinische Scores sowie klinische Parameter wurden im Rahmen der MR Untersuchungen mit der Zielsetzung erfasst neben der Validierung der Sequenzen eine Abschätzung der Effektgrößen für die klinische Forschung zu gewinnen.

1.2.3 Ergebnisse

Sowohl dGEMRIC als auch T2-mapping konnten zwischen Nativknorpel und Reparaturgewebe sowie zwischen Reparaturgewebe nach diversen chirurgischen Verfahren differenzieren. T1 und T2 sind einer hohen individuellen Schwankung unterworfen und müssen unter Berücksichtigung des Nativknorpel fallspezifisch interpretiert werden. Relative T2 Werte korrelieren mit dem klinischen Ergebnis, relative T1 Werte hingegen nicht.

1.2.4 Diskussion

T2-mapping sowie dGEMRIC können objektiv, reproduzierbar und vor allem non-invasiv die Ultrastruktur von Knorpelreparaturgewebe erfassen. Verschiedene chirurgische Techniken können gegeneinander differenziert werden. Unter Berücksichtigung einer Reihe von möglichen Fehlerquellen können mittels MR-mapping zusätzliche Effektgrößen zur Bewertung von knorpelchirurgischen Verfahren herangezogen werden. Die im Rahmen dieser Dissertation gewonnenen Daten zeigen, dass die Technologie das Potential zur Verbesserung der Effizienz klinischer Studien hat.

2 Introduction

2.1 Basic Cartilage Biology

Articular cartilage has a complex ultrastructure. Chondrocytes contribute less than 5% to the total volume; mechanical properties of hyaline cartilage depend on the extracellular matrix. Chondrocytes do not form cell-to-cell interactions but are embedded in the matrix. Changes in matrix composition as well as mechanical signals influence cell function [1, 2].

The 3 matrix regions (pericellular matrix, territorial matrix, interterritorial matrix) form a highly ordered network of collagen type II fibers that are linked to macromolecules of proteoglycans lined up on long filaments of hyaluronate. Small amounts of collagen types IX, X, fibronectin, decorin and biglycan are essential to the complex architecture of the matrix and not yet fully understood [1].

Change in composition between the joint surface and subchondral bone is described by dividing articular cartilage into 4 layers, or zones, referred to as: superficial, middle or transitional, deep or radial and the zone of calcified cartilage. Lamina splendens separates the cartilage from the synovial environment [1].

Differentiated chondrocytes are not able to proliferate. The lack of blood supply, of innervation and of lymphatic vessels, as well as the low mitotic activity and bradytrophic characteristics of chondrocytes contribute to a very limited ability to self-repair [2].

2.2 Cartilage Defects in the Knee

Healing of articular cartilage defects depends on the extent of the injury, the location in the joint, and the depth of the lesion.

Chondral defects do not elicit an inflammatory response since chondroprogenitor cells from underlying marrow do not have access to the injury and synovial cells are not able to adhere to the surface of injured tissue. Chondrocytes near the lesion create a response to injury, proliferating and synthesizing new matrix. However, chondrocytes do not migrate to the lesion and therefore are not able to fill the defect.

Defects reaching the subchondral vasculature show a very different response: approximately 5 days after initial fibrin clot formation, fibroblasts and collagen fibers parallel to the articular surface can be found. Metaplasia to cartilage finishes after several months, resulting in a fibrocartilaginous repair tissue. However, this repair tissue does not have the biomechanical properties of articular cartilage, and is unable to withstand joint loading long term. Subsequent degeneration often leads to a chronic, symptomatic defect, resulting in osteoarthritis and subsequent total knee arthroplasty [2, 3].

2.3 Surgical Cartilage Repair

Current repair options for damaged articular cartilage are limited. The current approaches in clinical practice are bone marrow stimulation techniques such as microfracture [4-7], osteochondral graft transplantation [8-11] and autologous chondrocyte implantation (ACI) [12-15]. Microfracture has been shown to be an efficient one-step procedure but produces mainly repair tissue, often with inadequate fill of the defect and limited loading capacity [16, 17]. Osteochondral transplantation or mosaicplasty is limited with respect to the size of the defect, unstable fixation and uneven surfaces in multiple grafting as well as cell impairment due to the mechanical forces during implantation [18]. ACI requires the excision of a periosteal flap to inject a cultured autologous cell suspension. ACI has been applied to more than 30,000 patients worldwide [15], however, cartilage overgrowth, delamination or fibrous degeneration of the newly formed tissue has been observed [19]. As a consequence, there is substantial interest in improving ACI. Biodegradable polymers based on

collagen [20-23], hyaluronan [24-26] or polylactides [27, 28] may allow a more predictable transport of the cells into the defect and may even promote chondrocyte differentiation [29]. These ACI techniques are often referred to as scaffold guided or matrix associated ACI (MACT).
Still, the question if there is a significant difference of repair tissue composition after different ACI techniques, has not yet been answered, and the efficacy of ACI in comparison with other techniques remains an issue of intense discussion [16, 30-32].

2.3.1 Mosaicplasty

Osteochondral autologous transplantation (OAT, mosaicplasty) is a frequently used technique and is suited for deep cartilage defects between 1 and 4cm^2, especially if the subchondral lamina is not intact [1]. Osteochondral plugs are taken from the non-weight-bearing areas of the femoral condyles with a cylindrical cutting device. Depending on the defect size, the plugs can be implanted as a mosaic to fill the defect and to restore the joint surface. Mosaicplasty is often an open procedure, although arthroscopic sets can be used. [9, 11].
The major advantage of this technique is that the defect is immediately filled with mature, intact cartilage. So far OAT is the only cartilage repair surgery which provides true hyaline cartilage. Disadvantages include donor site morbidity, limitation to defects below 4cm^2, lack of lateral cartilage integration with the penetration of synovial fluid and subsequent cyst formation, technical difficulties in the treatment of tibial defects and the technically demanding issue of the creation of a smooth and convex joint surface [18].
Hangody et al. [10] report 92% good or excellent results in a series of 597 femoral condyles treated with mosaicplasty, and other investigators report comparable outcomes [18, 33-35]. OAT certainly is an excellent treatment option if used in carefully selected indication.

2.3.2 Microfracture

Bone marrow stimulating techniques such as microfracture (MFX) are considered a good first line treatment for defects below 4cm² [1, 16, 17, 36, 37]. The technique was introduced by Steadman et al. [6] and can be applied during arthroscopy. After a careful debridement of the defect, the subchondral bone is penetrated with a pick (Figure 1). Microholes have to be deep enough to ensure bleeding from the bone marrow; however, the biomechanical integrity of the subchondral plate must be maintained. Subsequent bleeding and blood clot formation result in the formation of fibro-cartilaginous repair tissue. Improved knee function after microfracture is reported in 70 to 95% [6, 7, 16, 38]. Several studies report a substantial improvement 2 years after surgery [6, 7, 16, 38], but there are also reports of a decline in knee function after 18 months due to degeneration of the fibrous repair tissue [6, 36, 37]. Parameters related to successful cartilage repair with MFX are considered to be an age below 30 years [7, 16], a Body Mass Index (BMI) below 30kg/m² and a defect size below 4cm². Evidence was found that complete filling of the defect favors good clinical outcome [17].

Microfracture is a simple and efficient single step procedure and is a practical option for the first attempt of cartilage defect surgery, since subsequent treatment with ACI or OAT remains possible. However, the technique is, evidently, better suited for small defects, moreover young patients with large defects may profit more from ACI techniques in the long term.

2.3.3 ACI and MACT

ACI was introduced by Brittberg et al. in 1994 [13]. The technique is a two-stage procedure, and involves considerable complexity. During first look arthroscopy, a small piece of cartilage during biopsy is harvested. Chondrocytes are then enzymatically extracted from the biopsy specimen and expanded in monolayer cell culture. In the second stage, a periostal flap is harvested from the tibia, sewn over the defect, and finally, the cell suspension of expanded chondrocytes is injected into the chamber under the flap, which is terminally sealed with fibrin glue (Figure 2). ACI is considered a safe and efficient technique with good mid to long term results by several investigators [1, 12, 14, 15, 39-41]. ACI biopsy assessment demonstrated that repair tissue quality is subject to high variability [16, 19, 42-45]. Adverse events of classical ACI are predominantly complications related to the periostal flap: the occurrence of hypertrophy is reported to range from 2.4 to 20%, the overall need for further surgery varies between 5.1 and 37% [19].

The use of biodegradable scaffolds in matrix associated ACI (MACT) facilitates the surgical procedure since a periostal flap is no longer needed and cell delivery into the defect is ensured [3] (Figure 3). Three dimensional cell culture has been demonstrated to promote cell differentiation and the formation of hyaline-like repair tissue [29]. Biomaterials used in MACT are collagen [20-23], hyaluronan [24-26] or polylactides [27, 28]. The overall clinical results appear to be comparable to ACI with less morbidity and a lower rate of adverse events [24, 25, 30-32, 46, 47].

ACI is currently considered the best treatment option for large cartilage defects in young patients after trauma.

2.3.4 Cartilage Repair – comparison of surgical techniques

At this time, mosaicplasty is the only technique that can provide hyaline cartilage for the filling of osteochondral defects [3]. The implantation of osteochondral plugs is especially suited for osteochondral defects. The technique remains limited however, with respect to the defect size and donor site morbidity.

Microfracture appears to be a good option for the first line treatment of chondral defects if favorable clinical parameters exist (BMI, defect size below $2cm^2$, age below 30 years) [17, 36, 37]. Still, degeneration of the repair tissue and subsequent deterioration of knee function in the long term indicate that there is a need for improvement. ACI and MACT techniques seem to provide higher quality repair tissue, even though studies that compare ACI with alternative techniques show varying results. Knutsen et al. [16] did not find a significant difference between microfracture and ACI in the knee with regard to the clinical outcome at 2 years [16]. This also persisted at 5 years [48]. Horas et al. [49] favor mosaicplasty over ACI whereas Bentley et al. favor ACI [50]. Saris et al. report comparable clinical outcome, but better repair tissue quality in ACI in a randomized trial [51].

Still, with regard to the capability to cover large defects and the good to excellent long term results, ACI has gained a central role in cartilage surgery. It should further be emphasized that ACI is still under development and the full potential may not be achieved yet.

With regard to MACT, the overall clinical results seem to be comparable to ACI however with a lower rate of adverse events [24, 31]. Bartlett et al. [32] did not find a significant difference in clinical outcome 1 year after treatment with MACT vs ACI with a collagen membrane. Gooding et al. [52] found no statistical difference between the clinical outcome of ACI and ACI with a collagen type I/III membrane. Behrens et al. [30] report stable improvement in patients with matrix-associated autologous chondrocyte transplantation 5 years after implantation. Hyalograft C, an ACI technique guided with a scaffold based on hyaluronan, has also been demonstrated to provide comparable clinical results, even by arthroscopy [24-26, 53].

Kon et al. [54] compared Hyalograft and MFX in the knee in a prospective trial. Better clinical outcome was found after Hyalograft at 5 years. Sports activity level was comparable at 2 years but decreased at 5 years in microfracture.

The current treatment algorithm at the Department of Orthopedics, Medical University of Vienna, is as follows: Defects below $2cm^2$ are treated with microfracture under the condition that the subchondral lamina is intact. If the defect exceeds $2cm^2$ or if microfracture has failed, ACI will then be used, again under the condition that the subchondral lamina is intact or, in large osteochondral defects, that spongiosa plasty has been applied successfully. In osteochondral defects below $2cm^2$ mosaicplasty will be the treatment of choice.

2.3.5 Repair tissue composition and consequences for clinical application

Histologic reports on cartilage repair tissue quality usually grade tissue in categories such as 1 - hyaline, 2 - fibrocartilage-hyaline mixture, 3 - fibrocartilage, 4 - failure (inadequate biopsy, bone) [16, 25, 42]. The ICRS proposed to assess several morphologic criteria and gives a numeric score for biopsy assessment [55].

Reports on microfracture repair tissue composition indicate that the outcome varies considerably. Stromal cells of the bone marrow that are inducted into the defect through the microfrature have multipotent lineage capabilities that might lead to the formation of hyaline repair tissue [3], however the majority of microfracture procedures result in mixed fibrocartilage/hyaline or fibrous repair tissue [16, 51]. Fibrous tissue will not sustain the high biomechanical requirements associated with joint loading and as a consequence the process of degeneration starts, resulting in a decline of clinical outcome and may lead to osteoarthritis in the long term [37, 56].

ACI biopsy assessment demonstrates that repair tissue (RT) quality, similar to microfracture RT, is subject to a high variability [16, 42, 43, 51]. Henderson et al. [42] found hyaline or hyaline-like RT in 24 of 55 biopsies, 12 hyaline-like fibrocartilage and 19 fibrocartilage samples. In another study they found 9 hyaline or hyaline-like biopsies out of 13 [43]. Roberts et al. [57] report hyaline-like RT in 5 out of 23 graft patients. 11 cases had both hyaline and fibrocartilage morphology, 7 patients had fibrocartilage-like RT. Moriya et al. [58] found mixed morphology of hyaline cartilage and fibrocartilage in 4 patients, 2 samples showed fibrocartilage only. Mean glycosaminoglycan concentration of RT in 4 patients was significantly lower than normal, hyaline cartilage (NC).

With regard to MACT, data on histologic repair tissue evaluation remains scant. Gobbi et al. [53] report on 6 biopsies that were taken from the patella at an interval of 8 to 19 months after surgery. 4 samples were classified hyaline-like and 2 mixed fibro-hyaline. Marcacci et al. [25] report that out of 22 biopsies after 10 to 30 months 12 were hyaline, 6 mixed fibro-hyaline and 4 fibrocartilage.

With respect to the relation of repair tissue quality to clinical outcome, there is evidence that patients with hyaline repair tissue have better clinical outcome in the long term [42, 48, 56].

Nehrer et al. [56] evaluated repair tissue after reoperation due to failure and found fibrous tissue patterns with collagen X throughout failed cases. Henderson et al. [42] assessed ACI biopsies taken during re-arthroscopy after ACI and found that patients with symptoms unrelated to the cartilage repair procedure (Group A) had a higher rate of hyaline repair tissue than those with pain related to ACI (Group B). It was concluded that filling of the defect and thus coverage of the pain sensitive subchondral plate is the most important factor for pain relief in the short term whereas the durability of repair tissue and thus outcome in the long term will depend on repair tissue quality. Knutsen et al. [48] found after 5 years in a randomized trial comparing ACI and microfracture that there was no difference in the clinical outcome after either procedure and also found comparable rates of failure, however patients with hyaline repair tissue were less prone to failure.

In conclusion, the quality of cartilage repair tissue is subject to a high variability in all respective surgical techniques. Its composition is a determining factor for clinical outcome in the long term.

2.3.6 Repair tissue biopsy – aspects for clinical research

The invasiveness of the biopsy harvest leads to a very restrictive policy in histologic cartilage repair assessment. An extensive histologic evaluation of the wide variety of MACT techniques available seems beyond reach. The value of biopsy is additionally diminished by 2 other factors: first, a biopsy cannot be taken repeatedly to evaluate graft maturation over time. Second, a biopsy can only assess a small part of the repair tissue; in large repair sites with $10cm^2$ or more, a 2mm diameter probe may not be sufficiently representative for the repair site [51].
As a consequence, non-invasive, objective and reproducible parameters are required to assess cartilage repair tissue composition. MRI has the potential to meet these needs.

2.4 MRI of Cartilage

2.4.1 Morphologic MRI

2.4.1.1 Sequences

With the introduction of cartilage-sensitive sequences such as 3 dimensional gradient echo (3D-GRE) proton-density and T2-weighted (dual) fast spin echo (FSE) sequences with or without fat-suppression, the morphologic status of cartilage defects preoperatively and of repair tissue throughout the postoperative period can be reliably assessed. While 3D-GRE with fat suppression is suited to visualization of the thickness and surface of cartilage, dual FSE is sensitive to the internal cartilage structure as well [59-62]. This combination was recommended some years ago by the Articular Cartilage Imaging Group of the International Cartilage Repair Society [60, 63].

FSE imaging contrast is predominantly based on moderate T2 weighting and magnetization transfer effects. This results in low signal intensity of cartilage in contrast to the high signal intensity of joint fluid due to T2 weighting and the subchondral bone due to fatty marrow, which remains relatively hyperintense on FSE T2 sequences. Cartilage therefore appears dark against bright synovia and the subchondral plate [64, 65]. Intrachondral cartilage matrix damage and alterations of the cartilage surface can therefore be readily assessed. Another advantage of dual FSE is its inherent high resolution and low sensitivity to magnetic susceptibile artifacts, which are suppressed by the multiple refocusing 180° pulses of the FSE and allows reliable MRI assessment after surgery.

Standard T1-weighted fat-suppressed 3D spoiled gradient echo sequences provide a high signal intensity of cartilage while adjacent bone and synovial fluid remain dark. The 3D data set can be reformatted in any plane allowing 3D visualization and volume measurements [64, 66, 67]. New isotropic 3D-GRE sequences such as DESS (Double-Echo Steady-State), True FISP (Fast Imaging in Steady state Precession), Balanced-FFE (Fast Field Echo), VIBE (Volume Interpolated Breath-hold Examination) and MEDIC (Multi-Echo Data Image Combination), with a voxel size down to $0.5mm^3$ in the knee joint and $0.3mm^3$ in the ankle joint at 3T with a high gradient strength, have been developed and seem to be very promising for cartilage imaging [68-70]. 3D acquisitions yield even higher resolution and contrast-to-noise ratio than 2D acquisitions. Quantitative volume measurements can be added to cartilage assessment [61, 71, 72]. However, the integrity of these techniques has yet to be validated in clinical studies.

Rubenstein et al. [73] demonstrated that a resolution below 300µm is required to reveal fraying of the articular surface of cartilage. This finding stresses the importance of high resolution cartilage imaging. The

Introduction of high field MRI scanners into the clinical routine has considerably increased the possibilities of 3D imaging; GRE images yield high resolution in-plane and thin slices with a sufficient signal-to-noise ratio, while scan times can be kept well below ten minutes. New coil technology with multi-element design uses parallel imaging which has the potential to further decrease the scan time by a factor of 2-3.

In recent studies on cartilage repair, a 3D DESS sequence was found valuable for the first stage of cartilage assessment. The sequence provides an intermediate cartilage signal, high cartilage to fluid contrast and is suited for quantitative volumetric measurements [69]. The location of the defect or of repair sites can be defined and an optimal plane for further 2D sequences can be determined.

2.4.2 MR mapping

2.4.2.1 MR mapping – basic principles [74]

In diagnostic clinical MRI, the signal intensity (SI) of each pixel results from a vast number of intrinsic and extrinsic factors (Figure 4).

Extrinsic factors are defined by the MR unit properties (e.g. field strength, field homogeneity) and may be manipulated in the course of the examination (e.g. type of coil, sequence parameters, contrast agent). Intrinsic parameters are inherent to the examined sample (e.g. proton density, temperature, diffusion, perfusion) but may also be influenced by extrinsic parameters (e.g. T1 and T2 vary with field strength).

As a consequence, signal intensity is an unspecific, yet highly sensitive parameter. The diagnostic value of conventional morphologic imaging results from image contrast.

Fundamental image characteristics are:
- Image matrix: the number of pixels in x- and y-direction
- Field of view (FOV): image matrix size

- Spatial resolution: pixel size, resulting from image matrix and FOV size
- Contrast: the relative difference of signal intensity between 2 adjacent pixels
- Signal-to-noise ratio (SNR): signal quality, resulting from signal strength and background noise
- Contrast-to-noise ratio (CNR): influences image contrast; 2 adjacent pixels with differing signal intensity may not be distinguished due to high noise level
- Windowing: Attribution of SI to certain gray scale levels

The principle intrinsic parameters in clinical imaging are T1, T2 and proton density, which has lead to the terms T1, T2 and proton weighted images.

In contrast to morphologic images that are built of pixels with SI resulting from both intrinsic and extrinsic factors, pixels in pure T1 or T2 images (maps) reflect a distinct intrinsic parameter. Various gray or false color scales can be used to highlight patterns of damage in cartilage, however the main advantage of the concept is the ability to assess T1 or T2 in a distinct region of interest (ROI – mean T1 of the pixels assessed).

T1 can be assessed with an inversion recovery sequence. A 180° pulse initially inverts the proton magnetization and after a certain delay the inversion time (TI), a 90° pulse, is applied and the actual magnetization is read as a signal. The magnetization at TI will depend on T1. By the application of varying TI, T1 and subsequently T1 maps can be calculated.

In contrast to the inversion recovery sequence, a spin echo pulse sequence uses an initial 90° pulse to dephase the spins in the x-y plane. After a time delay τ, a 180° pulse is applied and at 2τ, that is defined as the echo time TE, an echo signal forms. If the 180° pulse is repeated, another echo with decreased amplitude (SI) will result. A multiple spin echo sequence thus can be used to calculate T2 through fitting of the amplitudes of the spin echoes.

Instead of a 180° pulse the echo can also be built up with the field gradients. Gradient echo sequences allow faster imaging and at 3T sufficient SNR and spatial resolution can be obtained with the use of dedicated coils.

2.4.2.2 T1 in cartilage

Based on pioneering work in articular cartilage research by Maroudas et al. [75] that demonstrated that fixed charged density of cartilage is related to glycosaminoglycan content (GAG), Bashir et al. [76] studied MRI imaging protocols to depict GAG. Under the assumption that GAG is associated with negative charge, Gadolinium Diethylenetriaminpantaacetic acid (GdDTPA^{2-}) will accumulate inversely to the GAG of cartilage. GdDTPA^{2-} alters T1. T1 weighted imaging protocols therefore were deemed to be sensitive for GAG content after contrast agent application [76].

After preliminary work in bovine and human cartilage samples [77] a comparison of intra-articular and intravenous application of GdDTPA^{2-} in human knee joints demonstrated that the intra venous (i.v.) GdDTPA^{2-} application was feasible to assess cartilage T1 [76]. An inversion recovery sequence was used that allowed quantitative T1 assessment and comparison with a T1 weighted morphologic sequence. Regions of osteoarthritic cartilage showed decreased T1 [76]. An interval of 45 minutes was found to be sufficient to ensure GdDTPA^{2-} distribution into femoral cartilage.

A subsequent study that compared the in vivo protocol with in vitro T1 imaging and histological assessment in patients after total knee arthroplasty confirmed that the technique could reliably assess cartilage GAG [78]. In vivo T1 and in vitro T1 values of distinct cartilage regions showed a strong correlation (Figure 5). Histological GAG assessment and post contrast in vitro T1 correlated whereas pre-contrast T1 did not. There was an excellent agreement of T1 and GAG distribution in MRI and histology. The sensitivity of post contrast T1 for cartilage degeneration exceeded morphological MRI and revealed enormous potential for the technique to assess early osteoarthritis.

Nieminen et al. [79] examined the correlation of spatial GAG distribution and T1 and concluded that absolute GdDTPA^{2-} determination might be prone to error, however the sensitivity of the technique to detect alterations in degenerated cartilage was confirmed.

Given that the pharmacokinetic properties of GdDTPA^{2-} significantly contribute to T1, factors that may contribute to GdDTPA^{2-} distribution in cartilage were examined [80]. It was concluded that (I) the dose would significantly influence the sensitivity, so double dose intra-veneous application in a concentration of 0.2mM/kg body weight was recommended, (II) that exercise after application was crucial to GdDTPA^{2-} distribution and (III) that the thickness of cartilage was determinative for the required length of the interval between application and measurement. The general protocol suggested double dose i.v. application of GdDTPA^{2-}, 10 minutes of exercise and MRI T1 measurement after 2 to 3 hours for the knee (due to patellar cartilage) and 30 to 90 minutes for the hip.

In summary, i.v. administered GdDTPA^{2-} enhanced quantitative T1 assessment can reliably visualize the GAG of hyaline cartilage. The imaging protocol has been established in literature under the name of delayed Gadolinium Enhanced Magnetic Resonance Imaging of Cartilage (dGEMRIC).

2.4.2.3 T2 in cartilage

The variation of T2 values across cartilage was first reported in 1989 and has been the subject of several studies since then [81]. T2 reflects the interaction between water molecules and water and surrounding molecules [81]. The interaction of water and collagen is at a minimum when oriented at 54.7° to the static magnetic field, which results in an increase of T2 (magic angle effect). As a consequence, the orientation of the cartilage collagen fibers to the magnetic field is reflected in T2, resulting in a spatial variation of T2 across cartilage that reflects the organization of the extracellular matrix. Nieminen et al. [82] compared polarized light microscopy and optical density of safranin O analysis with T2 in order to evaluate the morphologic parameters that determine T2 and concluded that proteoglycan content does not contribute significantly to T2, whereas the architecture of the collagen fibers is reflected in T2 through the magic angle effect. Free water and collagen content contribute to T2 as well.

As a consequence, in vitro investigations have been carried out to determine the magnitude of the magic angle effect. Grunder et al. [83] reported a 300% increase of T2 when the sample was oriented at 55° to the magnetic field. In MRI measurements in the knee, articular cartilage in the weight bearing areas will be oriented perpendicular to the magnetic field, whereas the cartilage of the posterior femoral condyle is oriented at the magic angle. Mosher et al. [84] questioned the relevance of this circumstance for in vivo T2 measurements in the knee and found that the magic angle effect contributed less than expected to variations in T2. At a normalized distance of 0.3 from the bone T2 increased 8.6% at 55°. At 0.6 T2 increased 18.3%, with the most pronounced near the surface with 29.1% at 55 degrees. However, at all orientations the zonal variation of T2 was clearly present (Figure 6). In conclusion, the increase of free water in the superficial zone during the absence of compression and conversely, a decrease of T2 of the superficial layer under compression was deemed to be more accountable for regional differences of T2 (especially joint loading areas versus the posterior femoral condyle) than the orientation to the magnetic field. The magic angle therefore is unlikely to account for the regional differences observed in clinical imaging.

As a consequence, T2 mapping has been widely applied in vivo MRI studies on osteoarthritis. Based on the hypothesis that the loss of proteoglycan will result in an increase of free water, increased T2 was expected to be a marker for osteoarthritis. However there is data demonstrating unchanged T2 or decreased T2 in degraded cartilage in vitro and in clinical T2 images [81]. A possible explanation is the creation of collagen cleavage sites in the course of degradation that interact with free water, decreasing T2. Wayne et al. [85] interestingly observed significant correlations between T2, mechanical properties and GAG content, suggesting that T2 might be sensitive to GAG loss. A decrease of GAG resulted in an increase of T2 and in a loss of mechanical stability which in turn decreased with GAG depletion. T2 was found to be a valuable indicator for biomechanical cartilage properties, however considering the T2 mechanisms mentioned above, a sensitivity to GAG seems to be unlikely. The increase of T2 may result from an increase of free water after GAG depletion, but is not specific to GAG loss. Increased free water and increased T2 will also occur through fibrillation and clefts in the course of chondromalacia.

The effect of age on T2 has been reported [86], however the range of individual cartilage T2 is such that case specific characterizations of cartilage properties can not be made. T2 may be regarded as an individual value that changes over time. Prospective studies on this question remain to be done.

As a consequence T2 is influenced by numerous factors in the course of osteoarthritis and can not be interpreted in a way that allows concise deductions to single causes of value alterations. T2 is presently not suited to monitor cartilage during trials on osteoarthritis. Rather, T2 is suited to assess architectural cartilage matrix properties or to study biomechanical cartilage properties in vivo.

2.5 MRI in Cartilage Repair

2.5.1 Morphologic MRI

Studies evaluating MRI in cartilage repair tissue monitoring had varying outcomes. Visual scores obtained in second look arthroscopies demonstrated a moderate correlation with MRI [43]. Tins et al. [45] found MRI did not correlate with histologic assessment, however, the MRI technique in their study did not meet the current level of MRI standards. Conversely, Roberts and al. [57] did report a significant correlation of graft histology and morphologic MRI. Watanabe et al. [44] examined the signal intensity and the development of T1 of ACI RT over a period of 36 months. T1 steadily decreased from high values after implantation towards the level of native cartilage after a period of 9 months. Most importantly, GAG content of RT was found to be significantly inferior to RC, which correlated well with the elevated T1 of RT. However, a direct correlation was beyond the scope of this study.

The undoubted value of MRI for morphologic cartilage repair evaluation has been demonstrated, and a wealth of information on morphologic cartilage repair criteria is reported in the literature [87-90].

2.5.2 Morphologic MRI Assessment of Microfracture, Mosaicplasty and ACI [89]

2.5.2.1 Microfracture

A recent study demonstrated MRI to be highly sensitive and specific in repair tissue assessment. Re-arthroscopy findings corresponded well with the pre-surgical MRI evaluation, even though a 1T unit was used. MRI specificity and sensitivity for defect filling were 100% and for repair tissue quality 80% and 82%, respectively [91]. MRI at 3T surely has the potential to further improve assessment [92, 93].

In a clinical study on MFX by Mithoefer et al. [17] MRI follow up was carried out with a 1.5 Tesla unit. 24 patients were assessed 12 +/- 2 months after surgery with parameters as follows: repair cartilage signal, lesion morphology, defect fill, peripheral repair tissue integration and subchondral edema.

With a cartilage sensitive FSE sequence [62], repair tissue signal was hyper-intense in 92% of patients. Mild subchondral edema was observed in 71%. Repair tissue fill was graded 67% to 100% in most cases; still, the majority had depressed morphology compared to adjacent cartilage. Osseous overgrowth occurred in 25%. Persistent gap formation at the border to adjacent cartilage was reported in 92%.

Interestingly, clinical improvement correlated with the fill grade ($p < 0.05$). Subsequent decrease of clinical outcome at 24 months occurred in all patients with a poor fill grade, and 3 cases with good fill grades decreased; moderate but significant correlations were found between fill grade and the activities of daily living score and the SF-36 physical component score. A lower body-mass index was associated with a better fill grade on MRI. Peripheral interfacing correlated well with the fill grade, but had no correlation with the outcome scores.

The filling grade of the defect would appear to be a major indicator of outcome of MFX; again, 3D GRE imaging at high resolutions may improve MRI assessment. Persistent gaps are considered adverse in MFX, and further investigation with larger numbers may be needed to determine if an association with repair tissue deterioration and subsequent failure in MFX exists. Mild subchondral edema apparently was not associated with clinical outcome; persistent alterations of the subchondral plate will also occur in long term follow-up.

2.5.2.2 Mosaicplasty

An MRI evaluation of osteochondral grafts should include: (I) the number and size of the grafts, (II) bone and cartilage integration, (III) the cartilage surface contour, (IV) an assessment of the signal in the graft, the adjacent bone marrow and at the donor site, (V) details of any soft tissue abnormalities and (VII) an assessment of the contrast enhancement patterns.

Cartilage and bone integration
Cartilage and bone integration should be considered separately.
Cartilage of the OAT was reported to be intact with regular surface in 85% of cases by Link et al. [94]. Gaps between OAT and native cartilage were rarely visualized with standard MRI. However, in indirect MR arthrography persistent fissure-like gaps between the implanted cartilage and native cartilage were demonstrated [95]. This finding corresponds well to OAT histology assessment and emphasizes the potential of contrast agent enhanced MRI in challenging cases.
Regarding the integration of OAT bone, cystic cavities with fluid-like signal intensity and/or a persistent oedema-like signal within the subchondral bone may be considered indicators for poor integration [94].

Cartilage and bone signal intensity
OAT bone marrow signal intensities are reported to be consistent with edema within the first 12 months after implantation (hypo intensity on T1-weighted images and hyper intensity on the fat-suppressed PD-w or T2-weighted images). During the 12 to 24 month period, a drop to 17% edema like signal intensities occurred [94]. Interestingly, among patients with OAT necrosis, T2 signal intensities varied depending on the morphologic type of necrosis (sclerotic or cystic degeneration). Clinical abnormalities were reported in only two of six patients with signs of OAT osteonecrosis [94]. Conversely, contrast enhanced MRI was specific to necrosis.
Sanders et al. [96] and Hangody and Fules [10] reported no cases of osteochondral necrosis in their patient groups.

OAT cartilage signal intensity is similar to the surrounding cartilage in the vast majority of cases [10, 94, 96].

Graft and adjacent bone

The early post-operative period is dominated by subchondral bone marrow edema, which resolves with graft incorporation. A normal fatty marrow signal is seen within and around the plugs when solid bony incorporation occurs [94-96].

Bone marrow edema can be expected in and around the grafts in approximately 50% of the subjects during the first 12 months. After this period, a gradual decline will be observed in the majority of cases; still, edema may persist in a small number of cases for up to 3 years.

Joint effusion and synovitis appear to follow a similar trend. Incongruities at the bone-bone interface occur frequently due to the variation of OAT and native cartilage thickness. The focus of OAT surgery is the congruity of the joint surface, and therefore is the main criterion in OAT integration assessment.

Complications assessed by MRI include graft loosening or migration, incongruencies of the cartilage-cartilage interface, significant gaps between osteochondral plugs and adjacent native cartilage and partial or complete graft necrosis. With respect to gaps, the post operative period has to be considered, since surface congruity will improve over time on account of fibrocartilagenous tissue formation between osteochondral plugs.

2.5.2.3 ACI and MACT

Assessment and interpretation of MR examinations for ACI and MACT patients should be performed in a systematic fashion. Careful attention should be paid to: (I) the degree of defect filling, (II) the integration of the graft to adjacent cartilage and underlying bone, (III) the grafts internal structure and surface, (IV) the grafts signal intensity, (V) any changes in the subchondral bone and finally, (VI), the presence of adhesions to the graft or joint effusion should be evaluated.

Defect filling

ACI repair tissue is chosen in order to have the same thickness as adjacent native cartilage, to restore the joint surface and to stabilize native cartilage. Filling assessment therefore concerns the thickness of repair tissue in 2D slices. Still, with 3D techniques available, repair tissue interfaces to adjacent normal cartilage can be assessed accurately in all directions and volume of the repair tissue may also be quantified.

Approximately 60 to 80 percent of cases after ACI can be expected to have complete defect filling [43, 45, 57, 97].

Graft hypertrophy, one of the major adverse events of ACI related to the use of a periostal flap, is reported to occur in 2.4 to 20 % of cases [19].

Graft hypertrophy is seen on MRI as the ACI graft protruding above the level of the native articular cartilage and may involve partial or the full width of the graft. Hypertrophy of grafts close to the intercondylar notch may cause impingement on the anterior cruciate ligament and requires arthroscopic debridement.

The incidence of graft hypertrophy after MACT is reported to be considerably lower and if present, may improve over time due to remodelling of the joint surface under weight bearing [24, 32, 97, 98].

Integration

The interface between ACI and native cartilage should be indiscernible. Splits or fissures at the border zone are considered pathological [87, 88] and are indicated by fluid-like signal clefts or ill defined high signal intensity at the interface in high resolution MRI [15, 87, 88, 99, 100].

The clinical importance of gaps in the integration zone lies in the possible progression to graft delamination. A thin rim of fluid between the base of the graft and the subchondral bone plate resembling a cartilage flap may indicate a delaminated graft still in situ at the repair site. A dislocated delaminated graft may appear as a loose body in the joint [87, 88]. Clinical symptoms are often pain, swelling and locking.

Structure & surface
Irregularities of the graft surface on MRI have been described previously in up to 50% of implants and thus seem to be relatively common during the first months after implantation [43, 66, 87, 88, 101]. At later stages, continuous smoothing of the graft surface has been observed, a finding that may be related to graft organization and remodeling. However, the development of surface defects over time is considered pathologic [97].
Graft tissue often has an inhomogeneous signal behaviour at early stages that differs from the trilaminar appearance of native cartilage. During the maturation progress, graft signal will become homogeneous in the majority of cases. Conversely, increasing heterogeneousness of the graft may indicate graft degeneration and beginning graft failure.

Signal intensity
4 weeks after transplantation the graft may have a fluid like appearance which could mimic graft delamination. However, on high-resolution imaging the surface of the implant is seen as a thin dark line. This feature is more commonly seen with classical ACI [87].
During the first 6 months after implantation, repair tissue signal intensity will differ from native cartilage; in the T1 weighted GRE sequence, signal will increase, whereas a decrease is to be expected in the FSE sequence [97, 102].
At 12 months, signal behaviour of repair tissue is reported to resemble native cartilage [43, 66, 87, 88] in the majority of cases in both sequences. There are reports of persisting hyperintensity in FSE up to 18 months. [103]. The exact role of signal intensity has not been determined yet, and may be subject to further studies.

Subchondral lamina and bone

The subchondral lamina is kept intact in ACI and MACT; however, in patients after osteochondrosis dissecans, defects of the lamina will persist after implantation. It is important to differentiate these cases from cortical endplate damage that occurs after implantation by overuse or recurrent trauma. Subchondral edema is reported to occur regularly within the first 3 to 6 months after implantation [43, 45, 87, 103, 104], and is part of the healing process. Persistence of edema after this period or even an increased intensity and size of subchondral edema should be considered abnormal and be closely monitored [87, 88, 105]. Edema may be caused by abnormal joint loading due to overuse or joint mal-alignment.

Cystic changes in the subchondral bone underneath the cartilage may indicate complications that require close clinical follow-up. Cyst formation have also been associated with a fibrocartilage, rather than hyaline-like, repair tissue composition [45].

Adhesions

Symptomatic intra-articular adhesions requiring arthroscopy occur in up to 10% of ACI patients. Aside from stiffness and pain, adhesions in connection to the Hoffa fat pat or the supra-patellar pouch can be a cause for graft dislocation by traction forces applied to the graft [15, 99, 100].

On MRI adhesions appear as bands of intermediate to low signal intensity that traverse the joint and originate from the repair tissue.

Effusion

Reactive synovitis is a cause of pain in the early postoperative period, but normally resolves. In cases of persisting effusion, alternate causes such as meniscal tears, ligament injury or the formation of new cartilage defects must be considered.

Regular development of ACI/MACT grafts

Serial MRI follow up of MACT patients demonstrated a dynamic healing process over time [87, 88]. Significant milestones of ACI and MACT repair tissue formation within the first year are: (I) Bone marrow edema can be expected in the first 3 months after surgery, but should recede afterwards. (II) The graft will have a fluid like appearance 4 weeks after implantation and then gradually approach the signal intensity of adjacent cartilage within 6 to 12 months. (III) Continuous graft remodeling, that may comprise gradual defect filling as well as intermittent graft hypertrophy, will result in complete defect filling with a smooth and intact surface after 12 months.

2.5.3 Morphologic Rating

The evaluation of the success of cartilage repair procedures [39, 106-110] requires specific grading systems, one of which is MOCART [97, 107-109]. The validity and reliability of this system has been evaluated for the assessment of matrix-associated autologous chondrocyte transplantation (MACT) in the knee [107], using 9 pertinent variables. These include filling of the defect, integration of the border zone to the adjacent cartilage, intactness of the subchondral lamina, intactness of the subchondral bone, signal intensities of the repair tissue compared to the adjacent native cartilage, and others. An almost perfect agreement between readers (ICC >0.81) was found for 8 of the 9 variables. When comparing the MRI scores with clinical outcome (knee related quality of life) 2 years after ACT, a statistically significant correlation was found for "filling of the defect," "structure of the repair tissue," "changes in the subchondral bone," and "signal intensities of the repair tissue".

2.5.4 T2 mapping – development in clinical use

Studies on T2 mapping and osteoarthritis yielded controversial results due to the complex mechanisms of the disease [81]. However, a basic condition for cartilage repair with microfracture and ACI is that the adjacent articular cartilage is intact. Under this assumption, T2 values of repair tissue can be compared to healthy cartilage in each patient, which substantially differentiates the application of T2 in cartilage repair monitoring from the application in osteoarthritis studies.

The majority of cartilage T2 mapping studies have used conventional multi-slice, multi spin echo (MSME) sequences, typically with a minimum of 7 echoes. The in vivo precision errors of the technique have been reported recently [111]. T2 provides a potential imaging biomarker of structural changes in the collagen matrix [112]. Increased cartilage T2 is associated with an increase in water content [113] and a decrease in collagen content [114] however the dominant factor influencing regional variation in T2 appears to be the anisotropic arrangement of the type II collagen matrix [82, 115-119].

A recent study observed a strong inverse correlation of fiber anisotropy determined with polarized light microscopy and the T2 of the cartilage [120]. The sensitivity of T2 to collagen architecture has been successfully utilized to study maturational changes in the collagen matrix of osteochondral plugs from juvenile animals [120-122] and age-related changes in mature cartilage [123-125].

2.5.5 T2 mapping – first applications in cartilage repair

T2 variation has the potential to provide very useful insight into the maturation process of cartilage repair tissue over time and facilitate a comparison with native healthy cartilage [116, 124]. Under ideal circumstances, cartilage repair tissue will develop a collagen network with a similar shape, collagen concentration and in particular a similar zonal organization as normal hyaline cartilage.

In a recent study by White et al. [126], normal hyaline cartilage and cartilage repair tissue were differentiated by zonal T2 mapping in equine subjects. Arthroscopic osteochondral autograft transplantation (OAT) and MFX were performed and evaluation of zonal T2 variation showed a characteristic distribution across the depth of the cartilage in control and OAT sites, with low T2 values near the subchondral bone and higher T2 values near the cartilage surface [126]. However no zonal variation was found within MFX repair tissue. Correlation with histology and collagen structural anisotropy as assessed by polarized light microscopy demonstrated a near perfect specificity of T2. OAT and normal hyaline cartilage sites illustrated a normal zonal collagen organization, whereas MFX showed disorganized fibrous reparative tissue was visible [126].

Using quantitative global T2 mapping of patients at different postoperative intervals after MACT surgery, significantly higher T2 values were found in cartilage repair tissue in the early stage (3–13 months) after surgery in an intra individual comparison with native hyaline cartilage [127]. Furthermore, a decrease in repair tissue T2 values was observed over time, with the T2 values becoming similar to native healthy cartilage. This finding was in agreement with a study by Kurkijarvi et al. [128] who, at 1.5 T, reported T2 values in the repair tissue and normal hyaline cartilage with 60 +/- 10 milliseconds and 50 +/- 7 milliseconds, respectively, in 10 patients at 10 to 15 months after ACI surgery. The zonal variation of repair tissue [127] has been demonstrated by the analysis of the T2 line profiles showing the variation of T2 values from the subchondral bone to cartilage surface. With increasing postoperative interval the shape of the T2 line profiles (and the calculated T2 line profile values) was found to become similar to the reference healthy cartilage sites [127].

2.5.6 T2 mapping – methodological studies

Spin echo imaging with separate acquisitions for each TE is considered a standard for T2 measurement, however not feasible in clinical routine due to acquisition time. Multislice multiecho spin echo (MESE) sequences provide faster imaging, but there are some aspects to be considered with regard to accuracy.

Multislice imaging requires slice-selective refocusing pulses that will produce transitional regions at slice boundaries. Resulting imperfect refocusing and thus stimulated echo contribution in fast spin echo introduce mixed T1 and T2 contrast to the image.

Furthermore, magnetization transfer contrast created by refocusing pulses for other slices diminishes signal intensity in cartilage and can thus impair the accuracy of T2 measurement [129].

Additional factors that may affect T2 quantifiaction are field inhomogeneities and insufficient sampling of the T2 decay curve [130].

Maier et al. [129] compared quantitative T2 measures obtained with a single echo spin echo sequence to multi echo T2 values in agarose phantoms with T2 values in the range of articular cartilage and differing T1 values at 1.5T. They found that T2 obtained with the multiecho sequence had an error of 10% that increased with longer T1. If however the first echo was dropped from the curve fitting, the error decreased considerably to 0.3 – 5.2%. The second and later echoes of the sequence had increased signal due to stimulation by the imperfect refocusing pulses. Elimination of the first pulse improved T2 accuracy because the decay rate of mixed T1/T2 was similar to pure T2. Comparison of the single slice spin echo sequence and multiecho sequence in volunteers confirmed that fitting of the second and subsequent echoes improved the error, however the error was still between -11.6% and 16.9%. Even though the qualitative T2 pattern of cartilage was comparable with the different sequences, absolute T2 differed considerably.

It was thus concluded that it may be very problematic to compare T2 values in literature when different T2 techniques are used.

Glaser et al. [111] evaluated the reproducibility of T2 in patellar cartilage and interestingly found a tendency toward higher regional precision errors for ROIs in the upper layers. Since their volunteer protocol was accurate (the four measurements were carried out each a week apart between 6 and 9 p.m. after one hour of rest) they concluded that partial volume effects deriving from the synovial fluid may cause more error than from the subchondral bone. However, the relative precision errors for T2 ranged between 2.76% and 5.37%, suggesting good discriminatory power of the technique. A study comparing T2 mapping at 1.5T and 3T demonstrated comparable coeffiecients of variation at either field strength in the same resolutions [131].

In light of emerging 3T scanners Pai et al. [130] conducted a comparative study at 3T of sequence dependent T2 quantification. Commercial T2 phantoms with different T2 values were measured with spin echo (SE), fast spin echo, multi echo spin echo (MESE), a spiral sequence and a 3D spoiled gradient sequence.

Interestingly, the MESE sequence had the best accuracy in phantom measurements. Subsequent in vivo measures in volunteers demonstrated in accordance with Maier et al. an increase in T2 measured by MESE compared to SE T2. With regard to the phantom study, the authors concluded that rather an T2 underestimation of the SE than an overestimation by the MESE was found in cartilage.

Reproducibility evaluation demonstrated coefficients of variance in the range of 0.1% to 2.8% in phantoms and 5.3% in cartilage in the MESE sequence; combined data an comparison with the other sequences showed that the average coefficient of variance was lowest in the MESE (1.3%).

However, all evaluated sequences demonstrated considerably different T2 both in phantom and in volunteers measurements. The comparison of T2 between different studies thus remains problematic.

2.5.7 dGEMRIC – clinical use

The dGEMRIC (delayed Gadolinium enhanced MRI of cartilage) technique, is currently the most widely used method for analyzing proteoglycan depletion in articular cartilage and has provided valuable results in vitro and in vivo [78, 80, 132-134]. Kim et al. demonstrated that global post contrast T1 correlated with the WOMAC Score in hips with developmental dysplasia [132]. A subsequent study demonstrated that T1 could be used as predictive value for the outcome of surgery; a threshold for a decreased probability of success after surgery was found at approximately 480 ms [135]. However, standard T1 mapping with inversion recovery is time consuming or limited to single slice acquisitions, as a consequence 3D applications of dGEMRIC that provide greater coverage and faster imaging times have been developed [136, 137].

2.5.8 dGEMRIC for the assessment of cartilage repair

In the evaluation of cartilage repair by means of dGEMRIC repair tissue shows heterogeneous T1 values compared to normal cartilage prior to the administration of $GDTPA^{2-}$, contrary to studies in normal or degenerative cartilage. Though post-contrast T1 mapping does not seem to correlate exactly with glycosaminoglycan content, the difference between pre- and post-contrast imaging (delta relaxation rate = $1/T1(Gd) - 1/T1precontrast$) does [138]. Watanabe et al. [138] demonstrated that the relative delta R1 index (delta relaxation rate of repair tissue divided by the delta relaxation rate of normal hyaline cartilage) correlates with the GAG concentration in repair tissue, as measured by gas chromatography, the accepted gold standard for the measurement of GAG content in biopsy samples.

Two other studies reported that dGEMRIC has potential as a non-invasive MR imaging technique for monitoring the GAG content after ACI [128, 139]. The findings of both studies suggest that the GAG concentration in repair cartilage at month 10 (or longer) after ACI is comparable to the GAG concentration in the adjacent normal hyaline cartilage. However the authors performed MR imaging only after intravenous contrast medium application and may thus have overestimated the GAG content in the repair tissue.

A recent study by Trattnig et al. [140] demonstrated that it is feasible to use a 3D variable flip angle dGEMRIC technique in patients following MACT surgery to obtain information related to the long-term development and maturation of grafts with clinically acceptable scan times. In accordance with Watanabe et al. [138] and Wayne et al. [85] this seems to confirm that pre contrast T1 has to be assessed for RT GAG.

In order to assess the maturation of cartilage implants over time, patients were subdivided into an early or late postoperative group (3 to 13 months and 19 to 42 months respectively) [140]. The mean R1 (in 1/sec) for repair tissue was 2.49 (±1.15) versus 1.04 (±0.56) at the intact control site in the early postoperative group, and 1.90 (±0.97) compared to 0.81 (±0.47) in the late postoperative group. The difference between repair tissue and normal hyaline cartilage was statistically significant ($p < 0.007$) in both groups, but the difference between repair tissue and normal hyaline cartilage between the groups was not statistically significant ($p=0.205$). The mean relative relaxation rate R1 was 2.40 in the early group and 2.35 in the late group.

2.5.9 dGEMRIC – methodological studies

For T1 measurements a 2D inversion recovery prepared fast spin echo at 1.5T has been established as T1 evaluation standard in cartilage in the course of the development of the dGEMRIC technique [136]. In order to evaluate the sequence for 3T and in order to evaluate a new, 3D inversion recovery spoiled gradient echo sequence a study on phantoms consisting of physiologic saline with different concentrations of GdDTPA was carried out.

Both at 1.5T and at 3T excellent agreement was found between the 2D and the 3D sequence. Even though acquisition time of the 3D sequence at 3T was 20 minutes, the advantage of T1 covering the whole joint was deemed worth the increased time.

Another approach on 3D T1 mapping is the use of a 3D dual flip angle technique [141]. Comparison between a fast 2 angle T1 mapping sequence (F2T1) and T1 mapping with an inversion recovery sequence (IR) at 1.5T in water/GdDTPA phantoms with different concentrations demonstrated high correlations of the T1 values. Multiple flip angles have been proposed in order to ensure precise measurements over a wide range of T1, however with regard to measurement time the dual flip angle approach was chosen and optimized for cartilage T1. A variety of different flip angle was evaluated and compared to inversion recovery T1 values. The combination of 4.8/26.9 degrees was found to yield the lowest mean error. Subsequent application in a patient series demonstrated significant differences, but still an excellent correlation of IR T1 and F2T1. It was hypothesized that slightly different ROI registration in the respective maps lead to the error. Still, an intrinsic weakness of the dual flip angle approach is that precise assessment is restricted to a relatively narrow range of T1 values. Flip angles have to be optimized for the respective applications.

The aspect of reproducibility is considerably more complex in dGEMRIC than in T2 mapping due to the use of contrast agent and its numerous associated biological co-factors such as diffusion, exercise after administration, renal elimination and cartilage thickness [80].

Interestingly, despite the wide use of dGEMRIC in clinical studies, data on the reproducibility are very limited. A first estimation based on measurements in five knees at two time points has been provided by

Burstein et al. who reported 10 to 15% error calculated as the ratio between the second and the first scan [80].

A recent study by Multanen et al. [142] evaluated the reproducibility of dGEMRIC in the knee at 1.5T by the means of the root-mean-square coefficient (CV) of variation and intra-class correlation coefficient (ICC). They carried out three scans in 10 healthy volunteers in average 5 days apart using the established protocol with double dose GdDTPA^{2-} and an inversion recovery sequence. A potential weakness of the study is that the FOV planning of the inversion recovery sequence in imaging sessions 2 and 3 was apparently based on the scout view. The T1 maps were aimed to derive from the center of the lateral condyle in the sagittal plane and from the patella in an axial plane. However they carried out very accurate region of interest analysis with 4 observers. The mean CV of full thickness ROIs was 7%, which can be considered a fairly good value considering the numerous factors contributing to post contrast T1. It is important to note that the ICC showed a wide range (0.61 – 0.96). This emphasizes the necessity of coherent and intense reader training. If ROI borders comprise subchondral lamina or synovial fluid, mean T1 can be altered significantly. This aspect was also represented in the fact that ICC values were better in thick cartilage areas.

In summary, the dGEMRIC technique can provide accurate and reproducible measurements if the numerous factors contributing to post-contrast T1 are taken into account, that is, if the imaging protocol is rigidly adhered to. Omission of exercise post-contrast, differing post-contrast intervals, errors in GdDTPA^{2-} dose, aberrant FOV planning and incorrect ROI analysis are main error sources that may bias the validity of the technique despite its high specificity for GAG.

2.6 MR Safety

Since the introduction of MRI to clinical use no persistent pathology has been reported directly related to the magnetic field [143]. Relevant effects like transient nausea, vertigo, visual effects or metallic taste may occur when moving in a strong magnetic field, yet pose no health risk and cease outside the field immediately.

Special consideration has to be devoted to implants. Especially stents and clips implanted before 1995 and long implants may develop considerable torque in high magnetic fields. Pacemakers and insulin pumps will malfunction in a strong magnetic field [143].

The gradient strength of a clinical 3T scanner is 40mT/m working in the frequency range of kHz; due to the linear increase of the Lorentz force with field strength, more noise will occur than at 1.5T. Sound intensity levels up to 132dB(A) can result, earplugs and headphones are thus mandatory during the exam. Furthermore the gradient fields may induce stimulation of muscles and nerves. Paraesthetic sensations, muscle twitch and visual effects can result, however clinical scanners have integrated safety protocols defined by the Federal Food and Drug Administration (FDA) and the International Electrotechnical Commission (IEC).

Due to the increase of Larmor frequency with field strength, radio frequency fields at 3.0T work in the range of 128 MHz for proton based imaging (high field, RF). Interaction with human tissue results in heating of tissue throughout body. Thermal receptors are located in the skin and patients may thus not feel a dangerous increase in core temperature. As a consequence, the FDA and IEC prescribe the integration of the specific absorption rate (SAR) into clinical scanners. It is a measure of the absorbed HF energy per kilogram body weight. It is worth noting that the RF pulse frequency contributes to SAR in a roughly quadratic ratio, SAR levels will thus increase by factor 4 if the field strength increases by factor 2.

Given SAR levels cannot be exceeded which precludes health risks under regular circumstances. The situation is different in patients with metallic implants. Even implants with low magnetic susceptibility such as Titanium can be heated significantly, especially if the length of the object is half the RF excitation pulse wavelength (approximately 13cm at 3T). Alternative imaging techniques may be preferable under such conditions [143].

Contrast agents based on gadolinium chelates have been introduced to clinical use in the 1980s and have been used in over 145 million MR examinations [144]. In 2006, first cases of nephrogenic systemic fibrosis (NSF) related to the use of MR contrast agent were reported. NSF has a mortality of 5%, however 30% suffer from severe impairment due to contractions, skin ulcera and limited range of motion. In May 2007, 255 cases of NSF were known worldwide. All cases had a significantly reduced function of the kidney (GFR < 30ml/min/1.73m^2).

The pathophysiological mechanism behind NSF has not been determined yet, however NSF apparently occurs in patients with severely impaired kidney function only [144]. In light of the long and widespread use of this MRI contrast agent, gadolinium chelates can still be considered safe if kidney dysfunction is screened for and considered before application.

2.7 Conclusion

T2 mapping and dGEMRIC have a high potential for non-invasive, objective and reproducible assessment of biochemical cartilage repair tissue composition.

Considerable effort is spent in clinical orthopaedic cartilage research on the evaluation of surgical cartilage repair techniques. Repair tissue quality determines clinical outcome, but is not easily determined due to the invasiveness of biopsy harvest. The efficacy of a new cartilage surgery technique has to be evaluated in the course of prospective clinical studies that require large numbers of patients and long term follow up (10 years minimum). If biochemical MRI can provide reliable data on repair tissue composition, a broad application in clinical research would provide a wealth of information that could shortcut the prospective evaluation of surgical techniques and thus considerably enhance cartilage repair research.

However, the introduction of new effect sizes into clinical research demands the evaluation of the feasibility in the course of studies and in clinical routine. Sequence validation and the assessment of preliminary values to estimate possible effect sizes will be required to determine reproducible and coherent examination protocols.

The aim of this thesis was to determine factors influencing the validity of MR parameter to characterize the clinical outcome after microfracture and MACT techniques on the base of several pilot studies.

3 Hypotheses

The prerequisite for surgical cartilage repair is that the adjacent cartilage is intact. In MRI, the repair tissue can be compared to normal, hyaline cartilage if no signs of OA such as osteophytes or significant thinning of cartilage are present. T1 and T2 mapping techniques allow for the assessment of cartilage ultra-structure and can differentiate between native cartilage and repair tissue.

The aim of this thesis was to evaluate how T1- and T2-mapping technologies at 3T available for clinical use can be used as additional effect sizes for the evaluation of surgical cartilage repair techniques.

The basis for the use in clinics was that both the T1- and T2-mapping techniques used would be accurate; therefore the reproducibility of the sequences was to be evaluated.

Considering the knowledge that exists from histological evaluations, the primary hypothesis was that T1 and T2 of repair tissue after MACT would differ significantly from MFX, and that the repair tissue after either surgical procedure would differ from native, hyaline cartilage.

Furthermore, the author hypothesized that repair tissue with T1 and T2 values comparable to the adjacent normal hyaline cartilage would be associated with better clinical outcome.

Finally, the author expected that T1 and T2 values would be in a dynamic range allowing for the definition of thresholds to differentiate between certain types of repair tissue quality and to gain additional information on the efficacy of surgical outcome.

3.1 Design

The design of the thesis is based on cross-sectional and non-randomized group and case series studies. The T1- and T2-mapping sequences were evaluated for reproducibility in phantom and in vitro cartilage sample measurement series. Clinical scores and parameters were assessed at the time of the MR examination in all studies and could then be used in a cumulative statistical analysis of the source data.

The case series have been summarized and are presented as follows:

I – all measurements and analyses concerning sequence validation measurements,

II – observational studies in patients to assess different types of repair tissue, and

III – assessment of the relationships between repair tissue properties in MRI and clinical outcome

3.2 Limitations

Harvest of histological samples in asymptomatic patients was beyond the scope of preliminary feasibility studies. Therefore histology was not available as a control in the respective studies. Cartilage integrity of the control sites was assessed with standard morphological MRI, however early stages of GAG depletion may not have been visible and thus introduced bias in the calculation of relative MR parameters.

Randomization was not feasible due to the strict cartilage repair treatment algorithm that is adhered to at the MUW. The MRI evaluation was not blinded with respect to the surgical techniques that were evaluated. However, MRI evaluations were blinded with respect to clinical outcome.

The non-randomized design of the patient groups may induce bias with regard to the clinical value, however this may be considered an intrinsic property of clinical pilot studies.

4 Methods

4.1 Patient Recruitment

All patients assessed in the course of this thesis were treated at the Department of Orthopaedics or at the Department of Traumatology at the Medical University of Vienna. Patient recruitment was carried out in the course of the clinical follow up in the outpatient clinic. Patients were invited to participate, and informed consent was obtained from all subjects prior to inclusion in accordance with the clinical study guidelines of the Medical University of Vienna.

Before the MRI examinations, all patients were evaluated with respect to MRI exclusion criteria and if contrast agent was to be used. Special care was taken to exclude the risk factors for the development of nephrogenic systemic fibrosis [144].

Morphologic MRI data were made available to the treating surgeons after evaluation by an experienced musculoskeletal radiologist to sustain clinical routine controls.

4.2 Cartilage Surgery

4.2.1 Microfracture

Microfracture was carried out as described by Steadman et al. [5]. During arthroscopy with a tourniquet, loose cartilage bodies were removed and marginally attached cartilage was debrided. After exact preparation of the bed, an arthroscopic 70° angled awl was used to penetrate the subchondral plate and to generate micro-holes in the exposed bone starting in the periphery of the lesion. Subchondral plate integrity was ensured by a minimum distance of 3mm between the micro-holes. After release of the tourniquet, bleeding from the perforations was ensured. A single drain without suction was placed suprapatellar medial in the outflow portal to reduce the risk of arthrofibrosis. The drain was removed 1 day after surgery.

4.2.2 MACT: Hyalograft C

Defects of the knee were assessed arthroscopically, and in case of a suitable defect, cartilage pieces were harvested during arthroscopy from a non-weight bearing area of the knee joint. Subsequent in vitro cell culture was carried out by Fidia Advanced Biopolymers, Abano Terme, Italy. After the enzymatic isolation from the extracellular matrix, chondrocytes were expanded in conventional monolayer cell culture for 2 weeks and then seeded on Hyaff 11, a hyaluronan based scaffold (Hyalograft C autograft). Hyaff-11 is a polymer of hyaluronan achieved by total esterification with benzyl alcohol that results in the formation of a three dimensional network of 20µm thick fibers that constitute a scaffold for cell adherence [47, 145]. The scaffold is biocompatible, insoluble in water, and undergoes a spontaneous process of hydrolysis, releasing benzylic alcohol and hyaluronan [146]. The polymer is sterilized by γ-irradiation, and is completely dissolved after approximately 4 months [147].

It has been demonstrated that cells redifferentiate to the chondrogenic phenotype in 3D cell culture and start to produce hyaline-like repair tissue in vitro [29]. 2 weeks after seeding, Hyalograft C autograft can be implanted in the defect site. The graft was delivered in a transportation medium, which permits application at least 72h after packing. However, the deep frozen biopsy specimen can be preserved up to 1 year after harvest, which allows for time to determine if a first line treatment like microfracture yields satisfactory improvement or if subsequent surgery is necessary.

Briefly, all patients underwent arthroscopy for cell harvest and were subsequently hospitalized for graft implantation 3 weeks or more post arthroscopy, as described above. Graft implantation was carried out by miniarthrotomy without a tourniquet in the majority of patients. The defects were carefully debrided, however during the implantation the integrity of the subchondral plate was preserved and the debridement performed thoroughly to achieve a stable adjacent cartilage. Then, defect size was templated with sterile paper, and the implant was cut to exactly fit the defect. Graft fixation was ensured with fibrin glue. Bleedings were stopped, and the arthrotomy was closed in layers without the use of a drain.

The arthroscopic implantation with a customized and patented instrument set which is very suitable for the treatment of anterior and central defects was used in 5 cases [26]. In standard arthroscopy, a Kirschner-wire was drilled into the defect site. The defect was milled with a front reamer up to the adjacent healthy articular cartilage without penetrating the subchondral bone. After that the water flow was stopped, the transplant was stamped out to the appropriate size, molded into the defect, and sealed with fibrin glue when necessary (Tissucol, Baxter, Austria).

4.2.3 MACT: BioCart II

BioCart™II is a biocompatible matrix (CartiMate™, ProChon, Israel) which is composed of processed plasminogen-free fibrinogen and thrombin, combined with small amounts of recombinant, non-crosslinked hyaluronic acid. It has a sponge-like 3D structure and provides a biodegradable, non-immunogenic scaffold which absorbs more than 90% of the seeded cells facilitating 3D distribution in their natural topology. A cartilage biopsy of approximately 150mg is harvested during first look arthroscopy. 140ml of blood are collected to obtain autologous serum for cell culture. Both blood and biopsy are sent to the GMP/GLP facility (ProChon Biotech Ltd., Nes Ziona, Israel) for chondrocyte isolation via enzymatic degradation in order to create a homogenous population of chondrocytes. The cell culture medium is supplemented with autologous human serum and a recombinant fibroblast growth factor 2 (FGF2) variant developed and provided by ProChon. The FGF2 variant aims to stimulate chondrocytes to multiply and also to maintain the capacity to re-differentiate and to produce hyaline-like RT once they are reintroduced to the patient. BioCart™II is assembled by seeding BioCart™ cells into CartiMate™ 3 to 4 days prior to the planned surgery. The approximate chondrocyte concentration of BioCart™II is 0.5×10^6 cells /cm^2.

Briefly, all patients underwent arthroscopy for cell harvest and received the graft 3 to 6 weeks later. Graft implantation was carried out by miniarthrotomy without a tourniquet. After careful debridement to attain stable adjacent cartilage defect size was templated with a sterile paper. The seeded BioCart™II implant was cut to fit exactly the defect and graft fixation was ensured with fibrin glue. Bleedings were stopped, and the arthrotomy was closed in layers without the use of a drain.

4.2.4 Rehabilitation

4.2.4.1 Microfracture

Postoperative treatment included continuous passive motion (CPM) for a period of 6 weeks after surgery. Crutch assisted non weight bearing ambulation was prescribed for 4 weeks and touch-down partial weight bearing up to 20kg for another 2 weeks. After 6 weeks patients progressed to full weight bearing, free or machine weights were not permitted before week 16. Sports that involve pivoting, cutting and jumping were prohibited until 6 months after surgery.

4.2.4.2 MACT

All patients obtained a brace immediately after surgery. Continuous passive motion started on the second day within a range of motion of 30°. Exercise continued until full flexion was achieved after 4 weeks. Crutch assisted non weight bearing ambulation was prescribed for 6 weeks. During post OP week 7 to 12 patients mobilized with touch down loading and finally progressed to free walking. After week 12 the rehabilitation program was no longer monitored. Moderate exercise such as short hikes or cycling was recommended 3 to 6 months after surgery. Sports that include stop-and-go and jumping were prohibited in the first year after surgery.

4.3 MRI

4.3.1 MRI Unit Specifications

MR examinations were performed on a 3T MR unit (Magnetom TIM Trio, Siemens Erlangen, Germany) with a maximum gradient strength of 40mT/m using an 8 channel (phased array) knee coil (In vivo, Gainesville, FL, USA).

4.3.2 Measurement Methods and Safety Considerations

Measurements were carried out feet first in supine position. The knee coil ensured a tight and stable positioning of the knee and also predefined joint flexion. Motion artifacts could thus be prevented fairly well. The middle of the coil was aligned with the joint line which was tagged with an erasable marker to ensure reproducible pre- and post contrast positioning.

All MRI examinations that were carried out in the course of the studies reported were subject to clinical routine safety guidelines. Patient assessment was carried out by a member of the medical MRI staff and by the physician responsible for the examination.

To rule out the risk of NSF, we employed the guidelines proposed by Michaely et al. [144] in our pre - MR examination protocol. In addition to routine clinical questions regarding claustrophobia, implants, tattoos and piercings, a questionnaire on NSF risk factors and recent (maximum 3 weeks) blood samples with serum kreatinine were assessed. NSF specific anamnesis included: diabetes, nephrotoxic substances, hypertension and chronic disease of the urogenital system (chronic infection and autoimmune diseases such as systemic lupus erythematodes, sklerodermia, glomerulonephritis).

4.3.3 Morphologic Assessment

The basis for morphological evaluation was an isotropic 3D-Double Echo Steady State (DESS) sequence with a TR of 15.1ms, TE of 5.11ms and a flip angle of 25° (Figure 7a). The field of view (FOV) was 150mm x 150mm with a 250 x 250 pixel matrix and a slice thickness of 0.6mm with an in plane resolution of 0.6mm x 0.6mm. An acceleration factor of 2 was applied; the scan time was 6min 32s.

This sequence has been introduced into clinical research in the course of a longitudinal follow-up study of the OA initiative to measure changes in cartilage thickness and volume and has been found to provide high precision in the detection of cartilage volume changes [148]. Additional evaluation in the femorotibial joint at 3T demonstrated even better results and reportedly permitted accurate and precise analysis of cartilage morphology [80].

4.3.4 dGEMRIC

4.3.4.1 Sequence

For quantitative T1 mapping a 3D GRE dual flip angle sequence, Volume Interpolated Breath-hold Examination (VIBE), with a TR of 50ms, a TE of 3.67ms, FOV 183 x 200mm and a matrix size of 317 x 384 was used, resulting in a resolution in plane of 0.6 x 0.5mm with a slice thickness of 1mm. One slab with 16 slices and a distance factor of 20% were applied. The bandwidth was 130Hz/pixel. The scan time was 6min 53s.

The sequence used flip angles of 10°/35° or 4.4°/24.7° both before and after intravenous administration of anionic gadolinium DTPA (Magnevist, Schering, Berlin, Germany; see Figures 7c and 7d). The post-contrast MR imaging protocol reported by Burstein [138] was followed. Post-contrast MR imaging was carried out 60 minutes after administration of the contrast agent. Careful identical positioning of the coil and knee joint and the use of 3 localizer sequences ensured the same slab orientation and location compared to the pre-contrast scan in each patient. Images were obtained in the sagittal plane.

4.3.4.2 Mapping Algorithm

3D dual flip angle (FA=α) T1 was calculated on a pixel-by- pixel basis j,k according to the equation:

$$T1c_{j,k} = \frac{TR}{\ln\left[\frac{\sin(\alpha_1)*\cos(\alpha_2) - Q_{j,k}\sin(\alpha_2)*\cos(\alpha_1)}{\sin(\alpha_1) - Q_{j,k}*\sin(\alpha_2)}\right]} \qquad Q_{j,k} = \frac{meas\_1_{j,k}}{meas\_2_{j,k}}$$

with T1c j,k = T1-value and Q j,k = quotient-pixel-values

4.3.4.3 Region of Interest Analysis

In each patient, 1 ROI was selected within the repair tissue (RT) and within normal reference cartilage (RC) on contiguous slices that covered the whole repair site in both pre- and post contrast maps. ROIs were identical in pre- and post contrast maps with respect to size and location (Figure 7c,d). Pre- and post contrast T1 values of RT and RC of contiguous slices were calculated to obtain global values. The author then calculated delta relaxation rates (ΔR1) of corresponding ROIs as follows:

$R1_{pre} = 1/T1_{pre}$ $R1_{post} = 1/T1_{post}$

$\Delta R1 = R1_{post} - R1_{pre}$

The relative delta relaxation rate (rΔR1) from ΔR1 of RT and RC was then calculated for each case [111, 130, 131]:

$r\Delta R1 = \Delta R1_{RT} / \Delta R1_{RC}$

4.3.5 T2 mapping

4.3.5.1 Sequence

The T2 relaxation times were obtained from T2 maps reconstructed using a multi-echo spin-echo technique with a repetition time (TR) of 1.650 s. Six echo times (TE) were collected (12.9ms, 25.8ms, 38.7ms, 51.6ms, 65.5ms and 77.4ms). A 200mm x 200mm FOV, 320 x 320 pixels matrix and a slice thickness of 1mm, with an in plane resolution of 0.6mm x 0.6mm and a distance factor of 100% was used. The bandwidth was 240Hz/pixel. The number of averages was 1 and the total scan time was 8min 46s. 16 slices were measured in the relevant compartment for each patient. Images were acquired in the sagittal plane.

4.3.5.2 Mapping Algorithm

Despite the influence of stimulated echoes within the echo train due to slice-selective refocusing pulses, associated imperfect refocusing and subsequently mixed T1 and T2 contrast, MESE sequences in proper configurations can provide accurate and reproducible T2 measurements [149]. The sequence used for the studies included in this thesis was optimized for cartilage imaging by Siemens Medical Solutions, Erlangen,

Germany with regard to the length of the echo train and number of echoes to minimize stimulated echo train contribution to T2.

T2 maps were obtained using a pixel wise, mono-exponential non-negative least squares (NNLS) fit analysis. The NNLS analysis has found wide application in T2 mapping of other body regions such as muscle [150] and brain [40, 151-156]. The algorithm is optimized to accommodate a noise floor and has been implemented to the TIM Trio MRI unit to permit online T2 map calculation (MapIt, Siemens Medical Solutions, Erlangen, Germany) immediately after the scans.

4.3.5.3 Region of Interest Analysis

Using morphological images and the intra-operative documentation as reference, slices covering the cartilage repair tissue were selected and region of interest (ROI) analysis was carried out. The ROIs were positioned within the cartilage RT and within a cartilage region that appeared intact (preserved thickness and surface, no signal alterations) on the morphological DESS sequence.

Special care was taken to avoid partial volume effects from the synovial fluid and the subchondral bone. For zonal variation analysis ROIs covered 50% of the full cartilage thickness (Figure 7b).

In each patient contiguous slices that comprised the whole repair site were evaluated. ROI mean values of all slices were then summarized and T2 of deep and superficial RT and RC was calculated.

ROI mean T2 and pixel number were then used to calculate global T2 values of RT and RC. In order to compare RT T2 of various patients, the author examined relative T2 values of the repair sites and of intact cartilage, respectively. The relative T2 (rT2) was calculated as follows:

$$rT2 = \frac{RT\ T2}{RC\ T2}$$

4.4 Clinical Evaluation

Several scores were used for clinical assessment, which included the IKDC Knee Form, the Subjective IKDC Knee Form and the Lysholm Score [151].

4.4.1 Lysholm Knee Score

The Lysholm Score was introduced in 1982 and subsequently modified for evaluation of ligament surgery [152]. It includes 8 sub-criteria, 3 of them functional and 5 subjective. A total of 100 points can be achieved, with 50% based on the symptoms of pain and instability, thus overemphasizing subjective symptoms. However, it has been demonstrated to be sensitive for chondral disorders of the knee [152, 153]. This score has a tendency to high outcome [156].

4.4.2 IKDC Rating

The IKDC form consists of a MODEMS TM compatible demographic form, a current health assessment form, a subjective knee evaluation form, a knee history form, a surgical documentation form, and a knee examination form.

The subjective knee evaluation and knee examination forms are essential to evaluation, whereas the other forms are added for convenience. Results are documented via verbal descriptions of normal, nearly normal, abnormal and severely abnormal. There are 4 categories used for evaluation, and 4 categories that are documented but not included in evaluation. The worst single value in a category defines the final result, thus making the IKDC knee examination a highly sensitive rating system. Persisting symptoms cannot be hidden behind high numerical scores related to other parameters [157, 158].

The subjective knee evaluation includes questions on pain and swelling of the knee joint, but emphasizes functional parameters as most of the questions are related to the level of activity patients can achieve. It has been demonstrated to be sensitive for ligamentous and meniscal injuries, patellofemoral pain, and osteoarthritis [159].

4.5 Ethical Considerations

The ratio of risk versus benefit can be considered favourable in MRI research (see section 1.6). If standard MRI safety guidelines are adhered to no additional risk will be associated with the cartilage specific MRI techniques. Patients may not gain immediate benefit from the examination, however the considerable gain of knowledge on cartilage repair may help to optimize the treatment of cartilage defects in the future.

All clinical studies carried out at the Medical University of Vienna have to be approved by the Institutional Review Board (IRB) which works in accordance with, and adheres to, the ethical principles for research including human subjects as stated by the World Medical Association Declaration of Helsinki.

IRB approval was obtained for all studies included in this thesis. The relevant protocols are registered at the Ethics Committee of the Medical University of Vienna (EK 355/2006, EK 93/2007, EK 358/2003).

4.6 Funding and Conflict of Interest

No conflict of interest exists with regard to affiliations with any organization or entity that had interest in the outcome of the respective studies. None of the authors were affiliated with stock ownership, employment or honoraria with the exception of Professor Avner Yayon, ProChon Biotech Ltd. who participated in writing the methods section of the manuscript 'T2 mapping and dGEMRIC of reparative cartilage after autologous chondrocyte implantation with a fibrin based scaffold in the knee: preliminary results'.

Project funding was mainly covered by the pre-existent infrastructure of the involved departments of the Medical University of Vienna. Additional funding was received by the FWF Austrian Science Fund, project numbers FWF-TRP-Project L243-B15 and FWF P 18110-B1.

4.7 Statistical Evaluation

Statistical analyses were carried out with SPSS 14.0 (SPSS Institute, Chicago, IL, USA) and Microsoft Excel on a Windows XP platform (Microsoft, Redmond, WA, USA) by the author.

T1 and T2 values obtained from the ROI analyses were processed by the means of descriptive statistics considering mean values, standard deviation, and the range (minimum – maximum). The ROI sizes (number of pixels) were considered to calculate the global values within a slice. The T1 and T2 values of repair tissue and reference cartilage are the mean of all slices assessed in each case.

For the phantom measurements, the ROI sizes were identical throughout all slices. The reproducibility assessment was carried out slice-wise, e.g. the ROI in slice 1 of sample 1 at time 1 was compared to the same ROI in slice 1 of sample 1 at time 2 etc. Reproducibility was expressed with the co-efficient of variation (COV).

In the evaluation of the VIBE sequence, the T1 values were compared to T1 assessed with the gold standard IR sequence; linear correlation analyses (Pearson) were used to determine the accuracy of the sequence.

Clinical baseline values were described using mean, standard deviation and the range (minimum – maximum). Mean values were compared using paired (if mean values from the same sample at different time points were compared) and un-paired student t-tests.

The relationship between clinical outcome and T1/T2 was evaluated with non-linear correlation analyses (Spearman's rho).

Further considerations of the relationship between repair tissue and reference cartilage T2 were assessed with linear regression fit analyses.

4.8 Study Plan

The data for this thesis were collected in a number of different studies; this was mainly due to patient availability and to focus on specific aspects in cartilage repair. Whereas the microfracture technique is quite common in orthopaedic surgery, the MACT techniques included were very new to clinics at the time of the data collection. In fact, the BioCart II cases were the first patients worldwide to be treated with this particular technique.

Due to the same MRI protocols applied the data of the various studies could be processed to gain further knowledge with higher numbers. The overall study design remained cross-sectional since all clinical studies were case series.

Although the MRI methods were the same for all studies (see sections 4.3.4 and 4.3.5), clinical baseline data of the patients assessed in the respective studies are given in the course of the results section. The overall study plan for this thesis is as follows:

4.8.1 Sequence Validation

2 separate studies to determine the reproducibility of the sequences used for the clinical studies were carried out.

The validation of the VIBE sequence (T1) included both phantom and cartilage specimen measurements that compared the accuracy and the reproducibility of the dual flip angle calculations.

The MESE T2 mapping technique´s reproducibilty was assessed both with agarose phantoms and cartilage specimens.

4.8.2 Case series to evaluate feasibility and range of effect sizes

The case series that could be assessed included:

- A consecutive case series of 8 cases after BioCartII (both T1 and T2)
- A case series of 10 cases after Hyalograft C (both T1 and T2)
- A cross-sectional series comparing 10 matched cases after MFX and 10 cases after Hyalograft with T2 mapping
- A cross-sectional series comparing 10 matched cases after MFX and 10 cases after Hyalograft with dGEMRIC

4.8.3 Correlation analyses of clinical outcome and MRI effect sizes

14 additional MFX cases could be assessed with T2 mapping. The source data of all cases were then used for correlation analyses and linear regression fit models to determine possible relationships between the MRI parameters and clinical parameters to characterize the value of T1 and T2 as effect sizes for clinical research.

5 Results

5.1 Sequence validation Studies

5.1.1 T1 - VIBE Sequence

5.1.1.1 Phantoms

The knee coil that was utilized in the patient series was used to evaluate T1 in 8 different phantoms consisting of saline solutions with varying concentrations of gadopentate dimeglumine (Magnevist, Schering, Berlin, Germany). The phantoms covered a range of T1 values between 200ms and 1250ms to cover the values expected pre- and postcontrast in human cartilage [127, 140].

An inversion recovery sequence at 7 non-equidistant TI times was used: 25, 75, 180, 350, 650, 1100 and 1680ms. Sixteen 2D slices with a matrix size of 256 x 256, a field of view (FOV) of 120 x 120mm and a 2mm slice thickness were measured. The bandwidth was 260Hz/pixel.

Subsequently, the VIBE sequence was applied and several different flip angle combinations were tested: 35°-10°, 37°-7°, 42°-8°, 46°-8°, 52°-10°, 61°-12°, 68°-13°, 71°-14° and 72°-15°. In an additional series, a flip angle combination of 24.7°- 4.4° was included. 3D GRE sequence parameters were as described above except for a matrix size 256x256, a FOV 120x120mm and an effective slice thickness of 2mm.

IR T1 maps were calculated with a non-linear two parameter LS-fit using IDL (RSI, Boulder, CO) software. The "MPcurvefit" IDL routine was used for fitting (Craig B. Markwardt, NASA/GSFC Code 662, Greenbelt, MD 20770; craigm@lheamail.gsfc.nasa.gov).

T1 maps were calculated with the algorithm described in section 4.3.4.2 and ROIs were drawn manually within each phantom and each slice, similar to the IR evaluation. Direct comparison of the T1 values from 3D dual flip angle dGEMRIC technique and IR technique was performed.

The best agreement between T1 in the IR sequence and T1 in the VIBE sequence was found for the dual flip angle combinations of 35°/10° with and 24.7°/4.4° degree combinations. The largest deviation of VIBE T1 was found in sample 8 (pure NaCl 0.9%).
More importantly, it was found that B1 inhomogeneity at the periphery of the coil resulted in a symmetrical alteration of the flip angles; therefore only the central 10 out of 16 measured slices had an acceptable agreement with the inversion recovery technique. The aberrance of the T1 values occurred in a symmetric pattern (equal deviations in slice 1 and 16, slice 2 and 15 etc.); only the central slices provided good agreement with IR T1.

The author carried out an additional measurement series of the 35°/10° and 24.7°/4.4° combinations to (1) assess the scale of T1 deviations to be expected in the peripheral slices of the slab, (2) to confirm that the T1 values resulting from the respective calculations were comparable to the T1 values assessed with inversion recovery sequence, and (3) to evaluate the reproducibility of the respective FA combinations. Furthermore, it was of interest if the T1 calculations based on the VIBE combinations could be improved if more FA combinations were considered.

8 phantoms consisting of different concentrations of Magnevist in saline solution were used: 1 – 1:200, 2 – 1:500, 3 – 1:750, 4 – 1:1000, 5 – 1:1500, 6 – 1:2000, 7 – 1:2500, and 8 – 1:3000. The author carried out the IR sequence and the 2 flip-angle combinations 35°/10° and 24.7°/4.4° with 22 slices.

The T1 times of each phantom were assessed by measuring 400 pixel ROIs throughout the slices of the slab both in the IR and in the VIBE sequences.

The difference between the T1 values in the VIBE sequences (T1-VIBE) and the T1 values in the inversion recovery sequence (T1-IR) were then expressed as a percentage of T1-IR in each slice for each phantom (-100 + (T1-VIBE/T1-IR)*100, see Figure 8). The mean differences for each slice were then calculated (Figure 9). The mean differences ranged from -19.2 to 12.8% in the 35°/10° combination and from -18.1 to 3.3% in the 24.7°/4.4° combination. As expected, the highest deviation was found in the peripheral slices. In the central 12 slices of the slab (slices #6 to #17), the mean differences ranged from -3.3 to 7.4% in the 35°/10° combination and from -4.0 to 3.3% in the 24.7°/4.4° combination.

Linear regression fit analyses were then carried out by the author to compare the agreement between the IR and the VIBE measurements. Using the values of all 8 phantoms in the central 12 slices of the measurement, excellent agreement was confirmed between the IR sequence and the VIBE sequences:

IR – 35°/10°   : T1 (35°/10°) =   -20.12 + 1.116*T1(IR), R^2 = 0.991
IR – 24.7°/4.4° : T1 (24.7°/4.4°)=   -1.67 + 1.013*T1(IR), R^2 = 0.993

Next the author tested the two flip angle combinations for reproducibility by 5 consecutive measurements in the 8 phantoms mentioned above.
The coefficient of variation (COV) of the 5 measurements was then calculated for each phantom.

Using the 10°/35° FA combination, the COV was:

    1 – 0.82%   5 – 1.46%
    2 – 1.46%   6 – 0.86%
    3 – 0.78%   7 – 1.17%
    4 – 0.83%   8 – 1.15%

Using the 24.4°/4.4° FA combination, the COV was:

1 – 0.69%
2 – 1.00%
3 – 0.92%
4 – 0.46%

5 – 0.51%
6 – 0.95%
7 – 1.29%
8 – 1.25%

An additional comparison of T1 was then carried out by (I) curve-fitting of the IR data in IDL, (II) by the pixel-by-pixel basis based on 2 FA combinations as used in clinics and (III) by curve fitting of the VIBE signal intensities using all 4 flip angles. The equation used was:

$$F = A(0)*\sin(X)*(1-EXP(-TR/A(1)))*EXP(-TE/A(2))/(1-\cos(X)*EXP(-TR/A(1)))$$

With $A(0)$ = the signal intensity, $A(1)$ = T1, $A(2)$ = T2 and X = the flip angle. T1 values were as follows (T1 values in ms, values from slice # 11):

Phantom #	IR	10°/35°	24.7°/4.4°	4 FA
1	927	1084	995	893
2	821	910	843	766
3	744	836	758	734
4	613	680	612	727
5	275	311	288	373
6	273	295	287	322
7	191	200	202	212
8	80	72	77	91
Difference to T1 in IR				
1		157	68	-34
2		89	22	-55
3		92	14	-10
4		67	-1	114
5		36	13	98
6		22	14	49
7		9	11	21
8		-8	-3	11

Linear regression analyses were used to compare IR T1 with the VIBE combinations; excellent agreement was found for all combinations:

R^2 IR – 35°/10°   = .998
R^2 IR – 24.7°/4.4° = .998
R^2 IR – 4FA   = .969

5.1.1.2 Cartilage Samples

In order to evaluate the sequence's sensitivity to B1 inhomogeneties in cartilage and to include magnetic transfer effects that occur in cartilage, the author carried out additional measurements in human cartilage samples in vitro using the same setting.

The samples were obtained from the lateral compartment of a patient undergoing total knee arthroplasty. As a consequence, the samples consisted of osteoarthritic and partly macroscopically altered cartilage. The samples were cut to fit in 20ml syringes filled with isotonic saline solution with a concentration of 0.2mmol/l Magnevist to simulate the actual in vivo conditions. To ensure complete CA diffusion, the interval between the preparation and the measurements was more than 12 hours.

The syringe containing the sample was positioned at the center of the knee coil and the cartilage layer was oriented perpendicular to the magnetic field. The sample was positioned at the center of the FOV.

Both the 35°/10° and the 24.7°/4.4° FA combinations were applied 3 times consecutively. The measurements were restarted after each series in order to make sure the MR unit calibrated for each measurement separately.

In each sample, 5 ROIs covering the cartilage were assessed. The ROI settings were repeated in all 3 measurements and care was taken to achieve equal positioning and ROI size (Figure 10 a-c). COVs were first calculated for each ROI series to account for the regional differences within the samples, and subsequently a mean COV was calculated for each sample.

The 10°/35° FA combination yielded T1 values as follows:

Sample	Measurement 1 (ms)	Measurement 2 (ms)	Measurement 3 (ms)	COV (%)
A	323 ± 21.4	327 ± 24.8	330 ± 24.7	1.68
B	370 ± 28.7	372 ± 22.3	377 ± 29.4	1.45
C	746 ± 25.9	754 ± 30.6	759 ± 30.8	0.95

The 24.7°/4.4° FA combination yielded T1 values as follows:

Sample	Measurement 1 (ms)	Measurement 2 (ms)	Measurement 3 (ms)	COV (%)
A	329 ± 27.1	333 ± 226.9	334 ± 25.5	1.17
B	375 ± 25.4	385 ± 27.4	381 ± 28.2	1.50
C	741 ± 28.4	742 ± 25.5	749 ± 26.5	0.79

To compare T1 assessed with the 2 different flip angle combinations, a linear bivariate correlation analysis that considered all 3 measurements (5 corresponding ROIs per sequence times 3) was carried out.

The linear regression fit was T1 (10/35) = -18.44 + 1.036 * T1 (4.4/24.4), R^2 was .999 indicating near perfect agreement between the 35°/10° and the 24.7°/4.4° VIBE sequences.

5.1.2 T2 Multi Echo Spin Echo Validation

5.1.2.1 T2 MESE validation - Phantoms

To attain data on the reproducibility of the T2 mapping technique, the author assessed three agar phantoms with varying concentrations (1%,

2%, 5%, agar in HBSS) with the 8-channel knee coil. Axial planes were assessed and ROI analysis was carried out in 6 slices in each of the 3 phantoms (1616 pixels per ROI); the measurements were repeated 3 times maintaining the exact same FOV planning in order to determine the coefficients of variance at the respective concentrations.

The mean T2 values (mean of 6 ROIs per measurement, 3 measurements) were:

Phantom	Measurement 1 (ms)	Measurement 2 (ms)	Measurement 3 (ms)	COV (%)
#1 (1%)	132.6 ± 2.58	136.0 ± 2.85	138.0 ± 2.52	2.50
#2 (2%)	83.7 ± 1.36	87.0 ± 1.60	89.4 ± 1.40	3.21
#3 (5%)	36.8 ± 0.34	38.3 ± 0.38	39.0 ± 0.29	2.49

These values are in the range reported in literature for MESE T2 mapping techniques [129-131].

5.1.2.2 T2 MESE validation - Cartilage Samples

The author additionally used the human cartilage samples that had been attained for the VIBE measurements to compare the reproducibility of the T2-mapping algorithm to the phantom measurements in the same session.

The 3 samples (A/B/C) were positioned so that cartilage surface was oriented perpendicular to B1. All samples were obtained from the posterior aspect of the lateral femoral condyle.

The measurements were carried out in the same knee coil used for the in vivo measurements. The T2 sequence was repeated 3 times with identical FOV orientations, and the on-line calculated maps were used for the ROI analyses. In each sample, 5 ROIs were placed that covered the complete extent of the layer. The ROI analyses were repeated for each measurement with manual ROI placement. The ROIs were oriented under consideration of morphological critera and size to achieve near-identical placement. In order to account regional differences of cartilage T2, the mean, standard deviation and COV were calculated for each series of 3 ROIs. Finally, the 5 COVs of each sample were used to calculate a mean COV of the sample.

The mean T2 values (mean of 5 ROIs per measurement, 3 measurements) were:

Sample	Measurement 1 (ms)	Measurement 2 (ms)	Measurement 3 (ms)	COV (%)
A	55.8 ± 14.00	52.2 ± 11.01	52.8 ± 13.97	6.54
B	49.4 ± 7.70	47.2 ± 4.55	50.0 ± 6.44	4.89
C	20.2 ± 5.72	18.8 ± 3.83	19.4 ± 5.55	7.11

5.2 Feasibility in vivo – observational case series studies

5.2.1 Overview of the Clinical Cases

Surgical Technique	Overall Number of cases assessed	dGEMRIC	T2-mapping	Lysholm Score at MR Examination
Hyalograft C	30	20	20	10
BioCart II	6	6	6	6
MFX	34	10	24	24

The clinical data included in this thesis derive from 5 studies, 2 of which the author took part in and 3 of which were carried out by the author as primary investigator; all patients that were managed by the author were assessed with clinical outcome measures at the time of the MR examination. The data of these cases were processed to the cumulative evaluation in section 5.3 of this thesis. The studies that were included in this thesis are:

[160]: Domayer SE, Welsch GH, Nehrer S, Chiari C, Dorotka R, Szomolanyi P, Mamisch TC, Yayon A, Trattnig S.
T2 mapping and dGEMRIC after autologous chondrocyte implantation with a fibrin-based scaffold in the knee: Preliminary results.
Eur J Radiol. 2009 Jan 19.

[161]: Welsch GH, Mamisch TC, Domayer SE, Dorotka R, Kutscha-Lissberg F, Marlovits S, White LM, Trattnig S.
Cartilage T2 assessment at 3-T MR imaging: in vivo differentiation of normal hyaline cartilage from reparative tissue after two cartilage repair procedures--initial experience.
Radiology. 2008 Apr;247(1):154-61.

[162]: Trattnig S, Mamisch TC, Pinker K, Domayer S, Szomolanyi P, Marlovits S, Kutscha-Lissberg F, Welsch GH.
Differentiating normal hyaline cartilage from post-surgical repair tissue using fast gradient echo imaging in delayed gadolinium-enhanced MRI (dGEMRIC) at 3 Tesla.
Eur Radiol. 2008 Jun;18(6):1251-9.

[163]: Domayer SE, Kutscha-Lissberg F, Welsch G, Dorotka R, Nehrer S, Gäbler C, Mamisch TC, Trattnig S.
T2 mapping in the knee after microfracture at 3.0 T: correlation of global T2 values and clinical outcome - preliminary results.
Osteoarthritis Cartilage. 2008 Aug;16(8):903-8.

5.2.2 Hyalograft C - 10 cases

5.2.2.1 Background and Aim

Hyalograft has been used in Austria since 2001, however data on the repair tissue quality remain sparse. The few histologic analyses published are promising, however not conclusive in terms of the actual efficacy of the technique [53].

The aim of this study was to evaluate Hyalograft repair tissue composition with T2 mapping and dGEMRIC to (I) provide additional data on Hyalograft repair tissue [24] and (II) to add cases for the evaluation of the relationship between T1, T2 and clinical outcome.

5.2.2.2 Study Specific Materials and Methods

The author assessed 10 patients with cartilage repair sites in the knee joint. 4 were female and 6 male, the mean age at implantation was 30 ± 9.5 (18 – 51) years. The mean Body Mass Index (BMI) was 24.0 ± 3.7 (19.1 – 29.3) kg/m^2. Lesions were located on the medial femoral condyle (MFC) in 9 cases and on the lateral femoral condyle (LFC) in 1 case. Mean defect size was 3.9 ± 1.9 (1.5 – 7.0)cm^2. All patients had deep defects, grade Outerbridge III-IV. The mean period from implantation to the first MRI follow up was 53 ± 22 range 24 to 80 months. The patients included in this study are part of a clinical prospective study on the efficacy of Hyalograft C [5, 16, 37, 42, 51]. All patients were treated at the Department of Orthopaedics, Medical University of Vienna in accordance with the methods described in section 3.

5.2.2.3 Results

At the time of follow up all patients reported knee function improvement: the Lysholm Score improved from 57 ± 12.8 before treatment to 90.4 ± 6.8 at follow up. Likewise there was an increase from 45.8 ± 23.9 to 71.5

±18.6 in the Subjective IKDC Knee Score. The difference was highly significant in both scores (P<0.001).

The IKDC Form was normal in 8 cases, nearly normal in 1 and abnormal in 1 case.

T2 values had a high variability both in RT and RC. Deep T2 was 39.0 ± 8.3ms (the range from 14 to 57ms) in RC and 42.0 ± 11.3ms (17 – 67ms) in RT, respectively. Superficial T2 was 42.4 ± 11.1ms (14 – 63ms) in RT and mean 44.2 ± 7.5ms (24 – 55ms) in RC.

Global T2 of RT and RC were 42.1 ± 9.0ms (18.9 – 52.2ms) and 42.1± 5.9 ms (28.9 – 49.5ms), respectively.

Paired double tailed student t-tests demonstrated a significant difference between deep and superficial RC T2 (p<0.001), whereas there were no significant differences between deep and superficial RT T2 (p=0.690). Global RT and RC T2 did not differ significantly either (p=0.996). rT2 was 0.99 ± 0.16 (0.65 - 1.16).

Pre-contrast T1 was 1513 ± 297ms (1051 – 2103ms) in RT and 1555 ± 287ms (1029 – 2142ms) in RC. Post-contrast T1 was 706 ± 194ms (435 – 1228ms) in RT and 968 ± 233ms (474 – 1455ms) in RC. The mean rΔR1 was 2.7 ± 2.5 (0.47-8.90).

5.2.3 T2 mapping and dGEMRIC of reparative cartilage after autologous chondrocyte implantation with a fibrin based scaffold in the knee: preliminary results [160]

5.2.3.1 Background and Aim

BioCart™II is a matrix augmented autologous chondrocyte technique that uses autogeneous blood serum to compose the matrix scaffold. The technique further combines the cells with a fibroblast growth factor variant to enhance the proliferation rate and aims to provide high quality repair tissue in patients with deep cartilage defects. The adverse events related to the use of a periosteal flap are avoided, and improved biocompatibility is expected as allogenic biomaterials are completely avoided.

This pilot study evaluated the repair tissue composition in the first patients treated worldwide. Both T2 mapping and dGEMRIC at 3T were available.

5.2.3.2 Study Specific Materials and Methods

Treatment with BioCart™ II was carried out in patients who met the following inclusion criteria: age 18 to 55 years, regular joint alignment, no signs of osteoarthrosis, intact ligaments and menisci, lesion size 1 to 8cm^2, lesion depth below 5mm and willing to undergo extensive rehabilitation.

The author obtained MRI of 5 patients with BioCart™ II between 15 and 27 months after implantation. 1 patient was treated in both knees (cases E and F), and all patients had deep osteochondral defects (Outerbridge grade IV) of the medial femoral condyle (MFC).

5.2.3.3 Results

At the time of follow up all patients reported knee function improvement: the Lysholm Score improved from mean 54.7 before surgery to mean 85.8 points at follow-up.

T2 values had a high variability both in RT and RC. ROI deep T2 mean was 45.4 ± 9.1 range 36.7 – 64.2ms in RT and mean 45.4 ± 8.3 range 32.0 – 58.9ms in RC, respectively. ROI superficial T2 was mean 48.0 ± 9.4 range 37.9 – 65.9ms in RT and mean 52.1 ± 8.6 range 41.2 – 68.8ms in RC.

Global T2 of RT and RC was mean 46.8 ± 8.8 range 38.4 – 65.5ms and mean 48.9 ± 7.6 range 36.8 – 62.5ms.

Paired double tailed student t-tests demonstrated a significant difference between deep and superficial RC T2 ($p=0.004$), whereas there was no significant difference between deep and superficial RT T2 ($p=0.148$, Figure 11). Global RT and RC T2 did not differ significantly ($p=0.307$). Relative T2 (rT2) ranged from 0.84 to 1.07.

Pre-contrast T1 was mean 1404.7 ± 339.6 range 1058 – 2223ms in RT and mean 1217.8 ± 174.8 range 865 – 1529ms in RC. Post-contrast T1 was mean 587.8 ± 299.9 range 231 – 1050ms in RT and mean 708.0 ± 226.4 range 438 – 1103ms in RC. Subsequently, a wide range in rΔR1 was found.

5.2.4 Cross-sectional cases series comparing Microfracture and Hyalograft repair tissue T2 properties [161]

5.2.4.1 Background and Aim

Based on the histological data available, microfracture was expected to result in lower quality repair tissue than Hyalograft; T2 mapping was newly available as an evaluation tool to directly compare cases after either technique.

The design of the study was a cross-sectional pilot comparing matched cases after microfracture (MFX) and matrix-associated autologous chondrocyte implantation (Hyalograft) to obtain first data on the differences in T2.

5.2.4.2 Study Specific Materials and Methods

20 patients (5 female, 15 male; mean age 40.5 ± 12.3, range 20 to 64 years) treated with MFX or Hyalograft (10 in each group) were included. Patients of both groups had undergone cartilage surgery due to single, symptomatic full thickness cartilage defects on the femoral condyle caused by trauma or osteochondritis dissecans. Clinical indication for MFX or Hyalograft was primarily based on the defect size. MFX and Hyalograft patients were matched with regard to age (MFX: 40 ± 15.4 years; MACT: 41 ± 8.9 years), defect localization and post-operative interval (MFX: 28 ± 15.2 months; Hyalograft: 27 ± 13.1 months).

Exclusion criteria were advanced or severe osteoarthritis, instability or deformity. Instability and deformity were excluded by clinical evaluation. In both groups the cartilage defect was located on the medial femoral condyle in 8 patients and on the lateral femoral condyle in 2 patients. The mean defect size for the MFX group was 2.55cm^2 (1.3 – 4.3cm^2) and for the Hyalograft group 5.34cm^2 (2.4 – 10.1cm^2).

The follow-up interval ranged from 12 to 64 months in MFX and from 12 54 months in the Hyalograft cases.

5.2.4.3 Results

The morphological evaluation based on the DESS sequence indicated no significant difference between patients after MFX or Hyalograft in terms of presence or absence of subchondral marrow edema, granulation tissue or cysts and joint effusion. Delamination, cleft formations or hypertrophy were excluded, however sclerosis of subchondral bone was more frequent in MFX. No significant difference between patients after MFX or patients after Hyalograft was observed.

The mean T2 values in control articular cartilage areas showed similar results in all patients (MFX: 57.8 ± 8.7, 40 – 66ms; Hyalograft: 56.7 ± 6.0, 50 – 67ms). The cartilage repair tissue in patients after MFX had a significantly reduced mean T2 value of 47.3 ± 10.3 (ranging from 33 to 64, p<0.05) relative to control tissue, whereas cartilage repair tissue in patients after Hyalograft was mean T2 value of 56.4 ± 9.6 (ranging from 45 to 72) and did not differ significantly from the control sites (p≥0.05).

Quantitative T2 measurements concerning zonal variation related to depth of articular cartilage showed differences between the control cartilage sites and the different cartilage repair procedures (Figure 12).

In the cases after MFX and after MACT, the reference cartilage sites had comparable T2 values, and the superficial zones had significantly higher T2 than the deep zones. In contrast, zonal repair tissue evaluation revealed that MFX RT did not have a zonal variation in T2, whereas MACT RT had T2 properties similar to the RC:

Technique	Site	Deep Layer	Superficial Layer	P Value
MFX	RC	53.7 ± 8.9	61.4 ± 8.7	< .05
	RT	46.4 ± 10.6	47.9 ± 10.2	**> .05**
MACT	RC	52.5 ± 6.0	61.0 ± 7.6	< .05
	RT	54.4 ± 9.8	57.0 ± 9.9	< .05

The clinical outcome assessed with the Lysholm Score was not significantly different between MFX and Hyalograft (p>0.05). In both cohorts, 8 cases had excellent and good, 1 patient fair and 1 patient poor outcome.

5.2.5 Differentiating normal hyaline cartilage from post-surgical repair tissue using fast gradient echo imaging in delayed gadolinium-enhanced MRI (dGEMRIC) at 3 T [162]

5.2.5.1 Background and Aim

The dGEMRIC technique had not been used before to assess differences between different types of cartilage repair techniques. The aim was to evaluate the relative glycosaminoglycan (GAG) content of repair tissue in patients after microfracture (MFX) and matrix-associated autologous chondrocyte implantation (Hyalograft) of the knee joint in a cross-sectional pilot comparing matched cases to obtain first data on the differences in T1.

5.2.5.2 Study Specific Materials and Methods

20 patients (5 female, 15 male; mean age 40.5 ± 12.3 years; age range 20 to 64 years) treated with MFX or Hyalograft (10 in each group) were enrolled in this study. The cases were matched in age (MFX: 37.1 ± 15.4 years; Hyalograft: 37.7 ± 8.9 years) and post-operative interval (MFX: 33.0 ± 5.2 months; MACT: 32.0 ± 13.1 months).

All cases had single symptomatic full thickness cartilage defects on the femoral condyle. The exclusion criteria were identical to section 5.2.3.2. In both groups the cartilage defect was located on the medial femoral condyle in 8 patients and on the lateral femoral condyle in 2 patients. The mean defect size was 2.55cm^2 (range: 1.3 – 4.3cm^2) in MFX and 5.34cm^2 (range: 2.4 – 10.1cm^2) in MACT.

5.2.5.3 Results

Different T1 values at the cartilage repair site compared to adjacent normal hyaline cartilage can be seen in MACT, even more so in MFX (Figure 13).

The mean ΔR1 for MFX was 1.07+/-0.34 versus 0.32+/-0.20 at the intact control site and for MACT 1.90+/-0.49 compared to 0.87+/-0.44 resulting in a relative delta relaxation rate (rΔR1) of 3.39 for MFX and 2.18 for MACT. The difference between the cartilage repair groups was statistically significant. In contrast, there was no significant difference in the Lysholm Score at follow up.

5.3 Correlation of T1 and T2 with clinical outcome

5.3.1 Methods

Both data available from the case series in section 5.2 and new cases were included; the Lysholm Score was chosen as clinical outcome measure because of its sensitivity for osteochondral symptoms.

Non-linear, bivariate correlation analysis (Spearman's rho) was chosen to evaluate possible relationships between clinical outcome and repair tissue properties. Linear regression fit analyses were used to consider confounding factors.

5.3.2 T1 – Cumulative Evaluation

5.3.2.1 Baseline data of the cases

Assessment included 24 cases. 8 cases had been treated with MFX, 6 with BioCart II and 10 with Hyalograft C. The mean rΔR1 was 2.80 ± 1.94 (0.47 – 8.9), age 32 ± 10 (15 to 60) years, BMI 24.2 ± 2.9 (19.1 – 29.1) kg/m², defect size 4.2 ± 2.1 (1.5 to 7.1)cm² and 89 ± 8.0 (65 – 100) in the Lysholm Score at MRI follow up. The number of cases was too low to allow for a conclusive correlation analysis stratified for treatment modality. The exclusion criteria comprised patients with trauma within the prior 6 weeks, recent intra-articular injections and knee arthroscopy within the prior 6 months as well as advanced osteoarthritis, ligament instability, genu varum or valgum malalignment and patients with no repair tissue in the site of defect. Lesions had to be localized in one compartment of the knee only. Patients' age was limited to 18 – 65 years of age and they had to be least 12 months post op. For single case data see Table 1.

5.3.2.2 Results

No significant differences were found between MFX, Hyalograft C and BioCart II with regard to age, BMI, defect size, rΔR1 and the Lysholm Score.

Spearman's rho did not reveal a significant correlation (r_s = 0.315, p=0.134) between rΔR1 and the Lysholm Score (Figure 14).

A moderate correlation between defect size and treatment modality according to cartilage surgery indication was found (r_s = 0.497, p=0.030). Treatment modality and rΔR1 correlated significantly (r_s = 0.512, p=0.011).

5.3.3 T2 – Cumulative Evaluation

5.3.3.1 Baseline data of the cases

The surgical treatment modality was microfracture (MFX) in 24 cases, Biocart II (Fibrin) in 6 cases and Hyalograft C (HYAFF) in 10 cases. The cumulative assessment included 40 cases. Relative T2 (rT2) was calculated for all cases for the correlation analysis. Mean rT2 was 0.91 ± 0.13 (0.61 – 1.16), age 37 ± 12 (15 to 65) years, BMI 25.8 ± 4.0 (19.1 – 38.3)kg/m², defect size 3.1 ± 2.0 (0.8 to 7.1)cm² and 83.8 ± 15.3 (36 – 100) in the Lysholm Score at MRI follow up. The exclusion criteria were the same as described in 5.3.2.1. For single case data see Table 2.

5.3.3.2 Results

In the independent samples double tailed student t-test, there was no significant difference between the Lysholm Scores of the respective treatment modalities.

Age, defect size, BMI and rT2 differed significantly after MFX and Hyalograft C as well as between MFX and Biocart II. There were no significant differences between cases after Hyalograft C and Biocart II.

Moderate correlations in bivariate non-parametric correlation analysis (Spearman' s rho, r_s) were found between the treatment modality and defect size as well as age (r_s = 0.655, p<0.001; r_s = -0.396, p=0.011), between age and defect size (r_s = -0.430, p=0.009) and between BMI and treatment modality as well as age (r_s = -0.400, p=0.011 and r_s = 0.530, p<0.001).

There was correlation of T2 in native cartilage with age (r_s = 0.5632, p<001) that fits very well with the data reported in literature. This did not hold true for repair tissue T2 (r_s = -0.216, p=0.180).

Bivariate correlation analyses (Spearman´s rho) revealed a moderate yet, highly significant correlation of rT2 with the Lysholm Score (r_s = 0.491, p=0.001, Figure 15).

There are also moderate correlations with the treatment modality (r_s = 0.470, p=0.002) and with age (r_s = -0.347, p=0.028). Linear regression analysis yielded R = 0.546 wit R^2 = 0.298. ANOVA testing of the model was significant (P = 0.005).

5.3.3.3 Stratification for the Microfracture Cases [163]

The 24 cases treated with microfracture had a mean age of 41 ± 14 years, 17 patients were male, 7 female. The repair site was located on the medial femoral condyle (MFC) in 19 cases, in 5 cases microfracture had been carried out on the lateral femoral condyle (LFC).

The mean defect size was 2.0 ± 1.1cm² (0.8 – 5.0cm²), the mean BMI was 27.2 ± 4.1kg/m², and the mean follow up period was 29 ± 14 months.

The filling of the defect was verified with morphologic MRI. Patients who had a filling grade below 25% of the defect size were excluded from quantitative T2 mapping analysis.

Mean T2 values of the repair sites ranged from 33 to 67ms (mean 49.8 ± 7.5), mean T2 values of normal, hyaline cartilage ranged from 40 to 71ms (mean 58.5 ± 7.0, Figure 16). A significant difference between T2 values was found in the paired, double tailed student t-test (p < 0.001).

Relative T2 (rT2) ranged from 0.61 to 1.02 (mean 0.86 ± 0.10) and was based on global ROI evaluations (Figure 17).

All patients reported improvement after surgery. The mean Lysholm Score was 80.6 ± 18.5 mean outcome of the Subjective IKDC Form was 70.0 ± 23.8. In the IKDC Rating, the knee status was normal in 41.7%, nearly normal in 45.8% and abnormal in 12.5%.

Repair tissue volume fill grade was above 75% in 66.7%. A range from 25 to 75% was found in 29.2%; in 4.1% filling grade was below 25%. Repair tissue hypertrophy did not occur in any patient in this study.

Moderate subchondral oedema was present in 1 patient.

rT2 correlated with the Lysholm Score (r_s = 0.641, p<0.001, Figure 18) and the IKDC Subjective Knee Evaluation Form (r_s = 0.549, p=0.005, Figure

19). There was no relationship between the IKDC Knee Form and the Lysholm Score (r_s = -0.284, p=0.179, Figure 20). Furthermore, there was no correlation of age, gender or the BMI with rT2 or clinical outcome.

5.4 Cartilage Repair Tissue Quality Assessment with T2 mapping

The correlation analyses confirmed a relationship between repair tissue with T2 comparable to the reference cartilage and good clinical outcome.
A linear regression fit model that compared RT T2 and RC T2 in each case should therefore be useful to give an estimate of the efficacy of the cartilage repair technique assessed.
Despite the limitations in terms of the number of cases available for a stratification for the treatment modality, it was considered of interest to calculate preliminary linear regression fits to explore possible differences (see Figure 21).

MFX (N = 24):   RT = 12.49 + 0.64*RT, R^2 = 0.35
MACT (N = 16):   RT = - 4.97 + 1.10*RT, R^2 = 0.71
    - Hyalograft C (N = 10): RT = -6.65 + 1.16*RC, R^2 = 0.57
    - BioCart II (N=6):   RT = -15.31 + 1.28*RC, R^2 = 0.82

6 Discussion

6.1 Overview

The primary goal of cartilage repair surgery is to fill the defect and to stabilize the adjacent cartilage. Complete covering of the subchondral plate appears to protect the sensitive nerval endings beneath the subchondral plate is a determining factor for short term outcome [1].

The secondary goal is to prevent the onset of osteoarthritis in the long term [42, 56], which is significantly influenced by repair tissue composition [42, 48, 51]. Cases with fibrous repair tissue are more prone to repair tissue degradation that will result in decreased defect filling and subsequently in destabilization of the adjacent native cartilage [131].

Current measures of cartilage repair outcome are clinical scores, morphologic MRI and histological analysis. Long term outcome can be evaluated only by the means of prospective, randomized trials that are associated with high costs and time or by histological analysis at earlier time points, which can save time, but is associated with surgery and thus not feasible repeatedly or in large numbers.

MR mapping has the potential to introduce new effect sizes that can considerably enhance the knowledge gained in the course of clinical trials. The cumulative source data evaluation of several MR pilot studies on cartilage repair demonstrates that both dGEMRIC and T2 mapping can differentiate between different types of repair tissue, are suited for in vivo cartilage assessment in the course of clinical studies and provide complementary information on repair tissue ultra-structure that is relevant for clinical outcome.

6.2 Methodological Considerations

The validity of absolute T1 and T2 has to be considered carefully. Both mapping techniques are subject to numerous factors influencing measurement accuracy and reproducibility.

Positioning and support of the joint during measurement is important to avoid motion artefacts and plays a major role for reproducibility. In T2 mapping, values will increase after rest due to water inflow into the weight bearing cartilage areas. The measurement should thus be preceded by a period of rest [130] or, alternatively, the T2 measurement should be carried out at the end of the examination. T2 measurement reproducibility can thus suffer considerably from varying measurement protocols.

Likewise, MR sequences must not be altered when assessing a study group. Pai et al. [130] compared different T2 sequences at 3T and demonstrated that 7 different T2 techniques yielded 7 different T2 values in phantoms with known T2. The errors were partly significant, ranging from -21.0% to 20.9%. Only the multi echo spin echo technique had a considerably smaller error (average -1.5%). Still, these data demonstrate that absolute T2 values obtained with different techniques, and even more so, with different MR scanners, can not be compared [140, 162, 164].

Similar considerations apply for T1 mapping with the VIBE sequence. Field homogeneity across the slices that will be evaluated must be ensured, and distortions must be accounted for in planning of the FOV. Even though the central slices yield T1 values comparable to those assessed with the inversion recovery sequence, the 3D dual flip angle approach on T1 mapping requires optimization of the flip angles for a certain range of T1 and careful planning of the FOV due to the considerable errors at the slab margins. The peripheral aspects of the volume assessed would not yield reliable data, only the central 50% can be considered for evaluation. This decreases the technique's efficiency considerably, as one can argue that almost half of the measurement time is in vain.

The flip angle combination is crucial for the accuracy of the mapping and should not be altered in the course of a case series [131]. It is important to note that the VIBE sequence has, being a GRE sequence, a particular sensitivity to magnetic susceptibility (e.g. abrasion wear after arthroscopy, haemorrhage after intra-articular infiltration). Inhomogeneties of B1 may result in altered flip angles, which will directly result in fitting errors and aberrant T1 values. This could be a problem in clinics as symptomatic patients will often have ongoing treatments or recent surgical intervention. In our case series recent infiltration therapy and arthroscopy within 6 months before the examination were therefore considered as exclusion criteria.

The curve-fitting algorithm will yield absolute values for each pixel, however the quality of the fit for each pixel is not reflected in the map. Except if a value resulting from poor fitting is obviously beyond the expected dynamic range, absolute values deriving from a poor fit would not be recognized and included in evaluation. Mapping values are thus considerably affected by low signal to noise and by artefacts such as motion and magnetic susceptibility (metallic abrasive wear after arthroscopy).

In the region of interest analysis, partial volume effects at the border of the cartilage layer are a particular source of bias, especially in zonal T2 evaluation. Synovial fluid may increase superficial T2 and be interpreted as zonal collagen organization instead of e.g. superficial layer fibrillation or disorganized cartilage matrix [84]. Despite unfavourable findings in in vitro studies, the magic angle effect has been found to be in a range that allows for T2 assessment at 3T [138]. Still, it should be noted that bias may be engendered if the repair site and cartilage reference region are not equally oriented to B_0.

In T1 mapping, ROI analysis is less prone to partial volume effects since global ROI analysis is performed and the cartilage borders can be avoided easily and obviously, there is no magic angle effect, which facilitates the choice of a reference site. Conversely, in order to obtain rΔR1, analysis has to be carried out in 2 separate measurements in the exact same ROIs. It is difficult to ensure the exact same positioning of the joint and the exact same slice orientation in 2 separate measurements. This intrinsic bias is further aggravated by the fact that measurement errors add up in the calculation of a coefficient. rΔR1 thus is subjected to a major source of bias, which has to be accounted for especially in light of the high specificity reported in literature [80].

The technique is additionally complicated by the use of contrast agent. The time interval post contrast has to be such that contrast agent distribution between the synovial fluid and cartilage is in equilibrium. If T1 is measured to early contrast agent distribution in areas with different GAG content may not be complete, whereas late measurement will be impaired by renal elimination of the contrast agent. Excercise after CA administration has been found to contribute significantly to complete distribution, and cartilage thickness determines the time until equilibrium. Protocols thus differ for each joint [142].

Multanen et al. [111] evaluated the reproducibility of dGEMRIC and found a mean error of 7%, however intra-class correlation between readers varied from 0.61 – 0.96, demonstrating that readers have to be thoroughly trained to achieve valid ROI evaluation.

The sequences used in the studies included in this thesis could be demonstrated to have acceptable reproducibility both in phantoms and in human cartilage specimens.

With regard to the VIBE, one has to account for the considerable distortion of T1 at the periphery of the slab; at the margin of the slab, errors in the range of 20% have to be expected. Still, acceptable correlation with the T1 IR sequence used as gold standard was demonstrated in the central 50% of the slab with a slight tendency towards higher T1 in the VIBE sequence. The FOV was increased accordingly, and only the central slices were used for the ROI analyses in the patient measurements. Since the cartilage repair sites assessed fitted easily into the central 50% of the slab, and the acquisition time was still relatively short, the T1 values assessed with the VIBE sequence can be considered valid.

Both the flip angle combinations of 35°-10° and of 24.7°- 4.4° provided sufficiently accurate T1 values in the long range of T1 of cartilage and repair tissue pre - contrast as well as in the short range of T1 values seen in post - contrast measurements. Still, a direct comparison of absolute IR T1 and VIBE T1 values to assess e.g. differences between stages of OA may be problematic.

Curve fitting considering 4 flip angles did not improve the accuracy in the phantoms. Particularly in patients, motion artefacts that will inevitably occur when measuring 4 flip angles, therefore the dual flip angle approach is the best option at this time.

With regard to the reproducibility of T2 mapping based on T2 multi echo spin echo, at 1.5T relative precison errors between 2.76% and 5.37% have been reported in literature demonstrating good discriminatory power [131]. Subsequent work comparing T2 mapping at 1.5T and 3T demonstrated comparable co-effiecients of variation at either field strength in the same resolutions [86].

The MESE T2 mapping protocol used in this thesis yielded excellent reproducibility in the phantoms with the COV ranging from 2.49 to 3.21%. In contrast, there were poorer results in the cartilage samples. It should be considered that the samples consisted of degraded cartilage and therefore had wide T2 ranges, which in turn affected the manual ROI evaluation. This did not play a role in the in vivo measurements, as the patients included had only intact or mildly altered (no loss in thickness, no fraying, no alterations in signal intensity) reference cartilage. The general application of the technique in vivo was easy as the measurement time was low, no contrast agent was required and the FOV planning based on the 3D DESS sequence allowed for a very exact placement of the T2 slab. The introduction of rT2 decreases the variation of values derived from different mapping techniques. Accuracy errors are thus evened out to some extent; conversely, relative values are subject of a biological source of error since integrity of the reference cartilage cannot be ensured. With regard to rΔR1 possible precision errors of 2 separate measurements have to be considered.

Additional difficulties for protocol standardization derive from the progress in MR research itself. New coil technology, new sequences, alternative mapping technologies such as T1rho [165-167], GAG CEST [168] or diffusion weighted imaging [29, 145, 146, 169, 170] and further increase in field strength providing higher resolutions and SNR yield ample room for improvement, but every modification can compromise the comparability with prior measurements. Any alteration of a given imaging protocol in the course of a study must obviously be avoided, or, if for some reason necessary re-validated.

In summary, absolute values obtained by MR mapping are prone to a number of potential bias-factors. In light of these considerations the characterization of cartilage repair tissue with relative values gains further importance. Even though bias might be introduced by impaired quality of reference cartilage, differences in the absolute T1 and T2 values due to technical issues can be evened out to some extent. Adherence to the same, strictly controlled MR protocols and ROI reading by trained readers are obligatory for the application of MR mapping in clinical research.

6.3 Case Series: Clinics and MRI

6.3.1 The case series in the context of clinical cartilage repair research

6.3.1.1 Hyalograft C

Hyalograft C has been found to have good biocompatibility, the potential to promote chondrocyte redifferentiation and to have suitable properties concerning biodegradability [24-26, 53, 54, 170, 171]. The data available from clinical studies is still limited, but investigators agree that Hyalograft C provides good clinical outcome and a low rate of failure and adverse events [53].

Histologic evaluation data on Hyalograft is very limited at this time. Gobbi et al. [25] report on 6 biopsies that were taken from the patella at an interval of 8 to 19 months after surgery. 4 samples were classified hyaline-like and 2 mixed fibro-hyaline. Marcacci et al. [127, 140, 161] report that of 22 biopsies at 10 to 30 months, 12 were hyaline, 6 mixed fibro-hyaline and 4 fibrocartilage.

The T1 and T2 repair tissue properties found in the current series agree with findings in prior studies [127, 140]. The mean rΔR1 of Hyalograft in prior study series was 2.15 and 2.35, respectively. RT in this case series apparently has lower GAG. Zonal T2 variation could be demonstrated in native cartilage, whereas it did not occur in repair tissue. RT properties found in this series are not as favourable as in prior series. Still, the close range of rT2 fits well with the perception that the repair tissue has a water and collagen content similar to the reference cartilage, contrary to microfracture repair tissue [172].

6.3.1.2 BioCart II

BioCart™ II has been introduced to clinical use very recently [127, 163]. This study provided the first data on the biochemical tissue properties of the repair tissue in vivo.

It is worthwhile to note that T2 had a high individual variability. There was a broad range of T2 values, which corresponded well with the results in the Hyalograft series and prior studies [140, 173]. The author found rT2 to be around 1, which indicates that RT collagen and water content was similar to that of the normal cartilage reference sites. T2 spatial variation of the RC corresponded well with the accepted knowledge about T2 zonal variation of articular cartilage. The increase of T2 was significant despite the low number of cases evaluated. Moreover, RT T2 also showed an increase towards the superficial layers, which indicated that the collagen ultrastructure of the RT resembled the RC reference sites (Figure 12).

In contrast, rΔR1 ranged from 0.77 to 4.91 resulting from a wide range of T1 in both normal cartilage and repair tissue. T1 of RT showed a higher variability than T1 of RC, which in consensus with prior studies [140, 173] lead us to interpret the wide range of rΔR1 as a variation of repair tissue quality in the respective cases. This agreed with the dGEMRIC analysis of the Hyalograft transplants [16, 25, 42, 53, 57, 58] and corresponds with the variability of ACI cartilage repair tissue reported in literature [172].

The foremost limitation of this study is the lack of histologic repair tissue evaluation. Another limitation is the number of cases available was limited due to the early stages of the technique [82, 126, 127].

It therefore is beyond the design of the study to characterize the efficacy of BioCart™ II for clinical use. Still, preliminary data indicate that the technique can provide high quality repair tissue similar to native, hyaline cartilage. Extended clinical research on BioCart™ II is indicated.

6.3.1.3 Microfracture versus Hyalograft C

T2 ranged from 40 to 67ms in the cartilage reference sites both in MFX and Hyalograft, the standard deviation was around 15% (MFX: 57.8 ± 8.7ms, 15.1%; Hyalograft: 58.7 ± 7.0ms, 15.5%). The repair sites had standard deviations in the range of 20% (MFX: 47.3 ± 10.3ms, 21.8%; Hyalograft: 56.4 ± 9.6ms, 17.0%) indicating the tissue was more heterogeneous than the reference cartilage. However, a cohort size of N = 10 was sufficient to draw statistically valid conclusions with respect to the differences in RT T2 of the 2 techniques: global repair tissue T2 in microfracture was significantly lower than in native cartilage. Lower MFX RT T2 can be interpreted as a consequence of lower water content in fibrous RT. T2 decrease over time was observed, even though the number of cases was too small for profound statistical evaluation.

In contrast, MACT RT T2 did not differ from native cartilage. This held true for both Hyalograft and BioCart II RT. Evidently, the RT had a water and collagen content closer to native cartilage than MFX.

Zonal evaluation demonstrated that MFX RT, as reported by several investigators, does not have an organized collagen network. In contrast to this, a zonal variation of T2 similar to native cartilage in MACT RT was found, though to a lesser degree and not in all the cases. These data to indicate that MACT RT collagen orientation can be similar to native cartilage.

T2 is not a specific parameter. The predominant value of T2 mapping lies in the assessment of RT ultra-structure organization. The technique may not be suited to assess single RT composition properties. The individual variation of T2 found both in native cartilage and in repair tissue lead us to use relative T2 (rT2). A case specific comparison of T2 in RC and RT was found to be important since the sole comparison of mean values can introduce bias.

The potential of T2 mapping to assess the organization of cartilage repair tissue and to differentiate between MFX and MACT repair tissue could be demonstrated.

A zonal variation of T2 across cartilage was found as expected [126, 127], and Hyalograft repair tissue had a zonal variation similar to hyaline cartilage whereas microfracture repair tissue did not in agreement with results of prior studies [1, 36, 37, 45, 100].

With regard to the GAG content in RT after MFX, biopsy evaluation data from other studies clearly show that the technique will mostly result in fibrous repair tissue that has lower GAG than native cartilage [128, 139].

The results of the series yielded the first data on the assessment of MFX with dGEMRIC. The rΔR1 was 3.39, indicating that the repair tissue had approximately a third of the GAG content of the reference site. This may be considered a poor outcome, however it agrees well with the histological data in literature and is conclusive. Like in T2 mapping, a sample size of N=10 yielded statistically significant results suggesting a good discriminatory capability of dGEMRIC in this application.

The mean rΔR1 found in the 2 Hyalograft series was 2.55 demonstrating the GAG content was higher than in MFX, however still far from native cartilage. The results after BioCart II show better quality (mean rΔR1=2.05, 4 of 6 cases had rΔR1 close to 1), but the range of rΔR1 reveals that the technique has a wide variability.

The reports in literature on ACI RT histology indicate that glycosaminoglycan (GAG) content is below that of native cartilage. Interestingly, early studies on dGEMRIC and ACI reported higher GAG content [16, 25, 51, 53], which may have been due to the lacking consideration of pre-contrast T1. With regard to the T1 data reported in the course of this thesis it is worth noting that the ACI techniques reported can not be compared to classic ACI, however the results agree very well with what is known from clinical trials and histological analyses [152, 153, 157, 158].

In conclusion, both MFX and MACT repair tissue had lower GAG content than native cartilage, and MFX resulted in even lower GAG than the MACT techniques. MFX repair tissue also had lower T2 indicating fibrous tissue with lower water content than articular cartilage opposed to more comparable RT T2 in the MACT techniques. Both techniques can result in very differing repair tissue quality, which is reflected by the wide ranges of rΔR1 and rT2 consistently found in all case series which agrees in turn, agrees with histological findings [16, 51].

6.4 Correlation of T1 and T2 with Clinical Outcome

6.4.1 T1

Both the Lysholm Score and the Subjective IKDC Knee Score have been demonstrated to be sensitive for osteochondral symptoms and were therefore selected for the bivariate correlation analysis of clinical outcome and RT composition [51].

In contrast to RT composition in MRI, there were no significant differences in clinical outcome after MFX and MACT. There was no correlation between the GAG content and clinical outcome.

This is in agreement with the results of the two large clinical trials comparing MFX and ACI by Knutsen et al. and by Saris et al. [16, 42]. Both investigators found at short-term no differences in clinical outcome despite the superior quality of repair tissue after ACI.

The major factor for the relieve of clinical symptoms is considered defect coverage to decrease mechanical stress on the subchondral bone [16, 48, 51]. In contrast, later follow-up showed in both studies that higher GAG content yielded better clinical outcome; in the cohorts of Knutsen et al., both MFX and ACI with higher GAG had better outcome at mid-term, however there were no significant differences between the cohorts. Saris et al. report the superior RT quality found in the ACI group results in significantly better clinical outcome at mid-term.

The current correlation analysis is a cross sectional view on a group of patients that is heterogeneous in terms of the follow-up period and lacks strength in numbers. As a result, the lack of correlation between rΔR1 and clinical outcome is in accordance with the results of the trials mentioned above [82]. A potential predictive value of rΔR1 for long term outcome has to be evaluated in the course of prospective studies, or by clinical follow-up of the subjects after 3 years.

The number of cases available for this evaluation does not permit a representative comparison of mean values. However there is a significant correlation of rΔR1 and treatment modality demonstrating that there is a trend towards higher glycosaminoglycan content in MACT repair tissue.

6.4.2 T2

T2 in cartilage has been shown to primarily reflect the zonal organization of the cartilage matrix and to be secondarily influenced by free water and collagen content [126]. A histological study in horses could demonstrate an excellent correlation of tissue organization between T2 maps and polarized light microscopy, both in cartilage and MFX repair tissue [86].

T2 map resolution obtained with the protocol described in the methods section allowed for a zonal evaluation of the knee cartilage. The increase of T2 in normal hyaline cartilage reported by other investigators was confirmed in our measurements. A wide range of T2 was found in healthy cartilage as well as a correlation with age, again, consistent with data reported in literature [81, 174].

The differences in age and defect size with respect to the modality of cartilage surgery were obviously related to the treatment indication criteria.

The correlations of clinical parameters showed a similar result. The significant differences in BMI between MFX and Hyalograft/Fibrin and resulting correlations can be considered as co-incidental bias resulting from the differences in age as the relationship between BMI and age is not related to cartilage surgery.

In contrast to this, rT2 differs significantly between MFX and Hyalograft C/Biocart II, resulting in a moderate correlation between treatment modality and rT2. The cumulative correlation analysis including MACT was consistent with the correlation between the Lysholm Score and rT2 found in MFX patients. Testing for confounding variables in multiple linear regression analysis demonstrated that rT2 has predictive value for clinical outcome even if age and treatment modality are taken into account.

In the MFX group, the minimum follow up period was 12 months to ensure mature repair tissue. BMI, defect size, age and gender did not correlate with clinical outcome. This may be due to the small number of patients examined. Defect filling did not correlate with clinical outcome either, however, patients without defect filling were excluded, so these results may not be representative for the MFX technique. Except for 1 patient, bone marrow edema was not present and thus was not evaluated in correlation analysis.

In agreement with the first series of 10 cases, it was confirmed that RT T2 was significantly lower than in native cartilage, reflecting the lower water content associated with fibrous RT [36, 37]. The mean follow-up period was 29 months. According to the findings of Kreuz et al. [152] RT can be expected to be fibrous by this time.

The Lysholm Score has been shown to assess functional impairment due to osteochondral defects [157, 158], and the IKDC Subjective Knee Evaluation Form is sensitive for ligamentous and meniscal injuries, patellofemoral pain, and osteoarthritis [111]. Significant correlation of both scores with relative T2 may indicate that repair tissue composition does influence clinical outcome. Conversely, criteria assessed with the IKDC Knee Examination Form are not related to osteoarthritis or cartilage defects, and the outcome of this form did not correlate with rT2 in the MFX cases.

Global T2 is a relatively non-specific parameter with regard to the contribution of numerous molecular mechanisms to T2. On the other hand, T2 appears to be highly sensitive for cartilage repair tissue function. The author found a highly significant correlation of clinical outcome in both the Lysholm score and the subjective IKDC Knee Score in patients after MFX. The MACT case series available for correlation analysis did not provide sufficient data for a profound intra-class analysis; however the cumulative evaluation confirmed the results of MFX analysis. Cases with rT2 around 1 (0.9 – 1.2) tend to have good-to-excellent clinical outcomes, whereas rT2 below 0.9 has an increased probability of poor clinical outcome. Multiple linear regression analysis with the Lysholm Score considering age and indication as confounding variables yielded an R^2 of 0.298. Considering the numerous factors contributing to the Lysholm Score not necessarily related to ostechondral disorders, this can be considered consistent, and rT2 < 0.9 might be used as a threshold value for RT function. However, randomized populations of both MFX and ACT/MACT patients have to be assessed to further substantiate this theorem.

In summary, dGEMRIC is not sensitive for clinical outcome however the potential as a marker for long-term outcome has yet to be evaluated. T2 has to be interpreted case specific in order to avoid bias related to the wide T2 range. Global relative T2 may help to estimate cartilage repair outcome in clinical terms.

6.5 Considerations on the Use of dGEMRIC and of T2 mapping in Clinical Research and Routine

Both dGEMRIC and T2 mapping can be implemented into clinical MRI easily from a technical point of view. There are no safety issues if standard MRI security is adhered to.

T2 mapping with satisfying signal to noise and resolution is feasible at 3T in measure times below 9 minutes and without the need of a contrast agent. Also, T2 maps provide a wealth of information.

It therefore appears advisable to implement T2 mapping in clinical MRI in all patients with cartilage repair in the knee at all follow up examinations.

In contrast, dGEMRIC is quite demanding in terms of time. Current data indicate both pre- and post contrast measurements are required. The interval between pre- and post contrast measurement to assess femoral cartilage in the knee has to be at least 60 minutes, which results in an overall examination time of over 2 hours. The necessity for contrast agent might reduce compliance.

Despite the valuable information gained with this technique, it therefore may not be suited for clinical routine imaging. However dGEMRIC is currently the only non-invasive technique available for clinical use to assess RT GAG content. Application in combination with T2 mapping might provide valuable data in prospective clinical studies on cartilage surgery. A multitude of ACI techniques has emerged and there is a pressing need to gain data on the repair tissue composition achieved. Aside from the difficulties associated with biopsy evaluation, most studies suffer from small numbers of patients due to the relatively low incidence of singular chondral defects. Multicenter studies therefore gain increasing importance. Quantitative MR mapping provides a tool for objectively and non-invasively assessing repair tissue composition. MRI measurements can be carried out in multiple centers and can yield equally valid data if the imaging protocols and MR unit specifications are harmonized. As a consequence MR mapping has a clear potential for the use in prospective multicenter studies.

Under the assumption that rT2 below 0.9 indicates an increased probability of worse clinical outcome than 1.0, a reasonable consideration of an effect size in the order of 0.1 seems appropriate, indicating more than 10% difference in RT T2 compared to RC T2. Assuming the COV of the T2-mapping technique used in this thesis (2.49 – 7.11 % in the phantoms and cartilage specimens), it has sufficient discriminative power to be used for the prospective assessment of rT2 differences.

Preliminary power calculation based on T2 MFX and MACT assessment [78] indicates that at power of 0.8, alpha 0.05 a sample size of 20 each is sufficient for significant statistical results in the comparison of repair tissue T2 (http://www.meduniwien.ac.at/medstat/research/samplesize/b2.html - 2009).

An estimation of the effect size of rΔR1 is not possible on the basis of current data. Longitudinal studies in larger numbers will have to be carried out to determine a possible predictive value and its relevance for clinical outcome. However, the reproducibility in post contrast imaging is reported to be 7%. There are no data available for pre-contrast, but the mean errors will add up. The discriminative power may be limited to assess differences greater than 10%. However, in the case series comparing MACT and MFX, the mean rΔR was 2.18 and 3.39, respectively, which is a difference of approximately 36%. The discriminative power of dGEMRIC to assess different types of repair tissue was therefore sufficient, but might not be good enough to distinguish between various MACT techniques.

In order to describe the efficacy of a cartilage repair technique using MR parameters, a linear regression fit model may be helpful; additional to the mean and standard deviation of rT2, analysis of the predictive value of the reference cartilage for the repair tissue can be characterized as follows: based on the assumption that good clinical outcome correlates with repair tissue T2 similar to that of native reference cartilage, and based on the individual variation of T2, one can expect that ideally, a cartilage repair technique should yield repair tissue with T2 identical to the native cartilage of the individual. A linear regression analysis of RC T2 and RT T2 would then yield RT = RC, which implies that k = 1 and e = 0 (RT = 1*RC + 0).

One could use k to describe the quality of the repair tissue, and R^2 of the linear fit to describe the reliability of the technique.

With regard to the T2 mapping results from this thesis, the different cartilage repair techniques can be described as follows:

MFX has a tendency to yield RT with lower T2 than the reference cartilage (reflected in the mean rT2 = and k = 0.64) and is not very reliable; RT T2 varies considerably (reflected in the range of rT2, or perhaps more accurately, in R^2 = 0.35).

Hyalograft and BioCart II provide RT more similar to RC (rT2 = 0.99 and 1.06, k = 1.16 and 1.28, respectively) and apparently are also more reliable (R^2 = 0.57 and 0.82) than MFX.

Particularly in T2 it might be problematic when the RT has higher values than the RC; an increase might be due to increased water content due to fibrillation of the tissue. The mean value and standard deviation can shadow outliers; in contrast, such would be reflected in a low R^2.

To give an example, looking at the 10 cases after Hyalograft, mean rT2 is 0.99, which may suggest that the technique yields RT almost identical to RC. The standard deviation is 0.16 (16.2%) which suggests an acceptable range. In the linear regression fit e = -6.65 and k = 1.16; both values indicate RT will be very similar to RC. However, considering R^2 = 0.57, one can say that the technique is not overly reliable. The chance for RT to have T2 comparable to that of the RC is only 57%.

In summary, the assessment of relative values can be recommended regarding the biologic factors and the relationship with clinical outcome, however to describe the efficacy of a particular technique one may prefer to carry out a linear regression fit analysis and give e, k and R^2 as additional effect sizes.

6.6 Limitations and Level of Evidence

The most apparent limitation to the interpretation of the data is the lack of histology. Both T1 and T2 assessment were based on the assumption that intact, hyaline reference cartilage was present to compare RT properties. Reference cartilage integrity was based on morphologic MRI. The main criteria were cartilage thickness, signal intensity, homogeneity, subchondral edema and cyst formation. Evidence has been found that a loss of GAG and disruption of the collagen network might not be reflected in conventional MRI imaging in early stages of osteoarthritis [175]. As a consequence, the integrity of reference cartilage was not confirmed by the means of histology and bias may have occurred with respect to relative markers. This is particularly true of dGEMRIC findings. If the reference region is depleted of GAG lower T1 will be measured post contrast and consequently rΔR1 will be closer to 1, indicating higher GAG in RT.

A 3D sequence was used both for pre- and post contrast T1 map planning to ensure exact congruent positioning, however it is worth to note again that the necessity of 2 separate measurements is an intrinsic weakness of rΔR1.

Similar considerations apply for T2; the technique has a better reproducibility since only 1 measurement is carried out and no contrast agent is needed. However, the magic angle effect further complicates the choice of the reference site and might bias values if the ROIs are oriented differently to the static magnetic field.

The levels of evidence of the studies that contributed to this thesis are 3 and 4, cross sectional studies and case series. All measurements lack histological verification, and present only a heterogeneous, one point in time view on a distinct group of patients. Since patient selection for MRI was subjected to the indication algorithm for cartilage repair surgery at the Medical University of Vienna, the results obtained may differ from randomized groups of patients. The findings discussed in this thesis have to be considered as pilot data for larger clinical studies. The results, however, do agree well with the existing knowledge from clinical research. They confirm that the inclusion of T1 and T2 parameters can improve clinical research provided the guidelines regarding how to use these techniques in clinical research are considered.

6.7 Outlook

The introduction of 3T scanners into clinical routine has yielded substantial progress in MR mapping, since the increased SNR has allowed higher resolutions in reasonable scan times. Still, there is a demand for further increase in field strength in cartilage imaging. In a study on canine cartilage Xia et al. [132, 135, 176, 177] provided preliminary in vitro data on T2 mapping at 7T with 13.7µm in plane pixel resolution maps. PLM verified line profiles that corresponded with the histological zones of cartilage in the very thin cartilage samples. These data show a considerable potential for the improvement of T2 mapping at 3T. The current resolutions may suffice for the thick cartilage layers of the knee, however do not allow zonal evaluation of hip cartilage or of talar cartilage, even though there is considerable interest in orthopedic surgery to do so.
Likewise, preliminary dGEMRIC analysis of the first carpometacarpal joint and dGEMRIC analysis of the hip show that the technique may have considerable impact in the clinical research, but will require higher resolutions to assess thin cartilage layers and to reliably separate cartilages of corresponding joint bearing areas [178].
The first in vivo measurements at 7T both in volunteers and patients after Hyalograft confirmed this notion [179]. T2 map in plane resolutions of

0.42x0.42mm were achieved, and T1 map resolutions were improved to 0.39x0.39mm.

Preliminary data in the patient case series demonstrated the expected zonal variation of native cartilage and a less pronounced, but still obvious increase of T2 towards the repair tissue surface. Interestingly, the range of T2 was slightly increased in comparison to 3T. T1 however was longer than at 3T (1259±277 range 909 to 2002ms pre-contrast and 683±141 range 404 to 1072ms post contrast). Higher spatial resolution and enhanced contrast at 7T thus may yield even more information on cartilage ultra-structure than current techniques.

Another important step for clinical use will be to determine the predictive value of T1 and T2 for the long-term clinical outcome. Similar to the use of histology, a possible study design comprises of further clinical follow-up and re-evaluation of the MRI data at later time points. For dGEMRIC at 1.5T, this has been carried out in the hip; dGEMRIC was demonstrated to have a predicitive value for the rate of failure after periacetabular osteotomy in dysplasia [135].

6.8 Conclusion

The results obtained in this thesis show that cartilage repair monitoring can be substantially enhanced by the implementation of dGEMRIC and T2 mapping into clinical trials.

The sequences were evaluated for their reproducibility and were found to provide sufficient accuracy albeit a number of intrinsic methodological weaknesses, which need to be considered in evaluation. Rigid imaging protocols and evaluation by expert readers are therefore basic conditions for the application in clinical research. The absolute values obtained in MR mapping are prone to a number of bias sources that can substantially impair the validity of the methods, therefore relative values should be used.

The pilot studies showed that both dGEMRIC and T2 mapping were feasible in a clinical setting and that the first results agreed with the histologic data on cartilage repair tissue quality available at this time. The techniques are suited for the implementation into clinical studies, complement each other, provide good sensitivity for the differentiation of repair tissue and confer data on cartilage repair tissue ultra-structure that have relevance for the clinical outcome.

The cumulative evaluation of the 4 pilot studies revealed that rT2 correlated with the clinical outcome and that a linear regression fit model is suited to characterize cartilage repair techniques.

Further prospective studies in larger numbers are justified to evaluate the predictive value of the MR parameters for clinical outcome.

7 Tables

Unit	Case #	rΔR1	Lysholm	Modality	BMI kg/m²	Defsize cm²	Age years	Sex
	1	3.54	86	MFX	27.1	1.5	40	m
	2	2.62	91	MFX	21.6	2.3	41	m
	3	2.48	100	MFX	24.6	2.6	42	m
	4	5.67	90	MFX	29.4	3	60	m
	5	4.66	65	MFX	22.7	2	36	m
	6	3.78	95	MFX	24.0	2.5	17	m
	7	2.25	95	MFX	24.3	4.5	41	m
	8	3.41	95	MFX	24.5	5	15	m
	9	1.14	91	Hyalograft	27.8	3	27	m
	10	2.1	100	Hyalograft	23.7	4	29	m
	11	3.1	92	Hyalograft	23.6	2.5	51	f
	12	4.92	94	Hyalograft	22.0	7	39	m
	13	1.67	76	Hyalograft	28.7	3	28	f
	14	1.95	90	Hyalograft	19.1	1.5	21	f
	15	1.02	82	Hyalograft	20.8	1.5	32	f
	16	0.47	90	Hyalograft	19.6	6	19	m
	17	8.9	94	Hyalograft	25.0	6	32	m
	18	1.92	95	Hyalograft	29.3	4	25	m
	19	1.42	85	BioCart II	23.2	3.1	38	m
	20	0.77	90	BioCart II	20.6	3.1	30	m
	21	0.87	75	BioCart II	21.3	7.1	27	m
	22	2.05	85	BioCart II	24.3	7.1	40	m
	23	1.57	90	BioCart II	25.5	4.9	31	m
	24	4.91	90	BioCart II	25.5	7.1	32	m
Mean		2.80	89.0		24.09	3.93	33.06	
STD		1.94	8.05		2.91	1.92	10.60	
MIN		0.47	65		19.1	1.5	15	
MAX		8.90	100		29.4	7.1	60	

Table 1: Single case table of relative delta relaxation rate and clinical parameters – correlation analysis source data

Case #	RT T2	RC T2	rT2	Lysholm	Modality	BMI	Defect	Age	Sex
Unit	ms	ms				kg/m^2	cm^2	years	
1	36	50	0.72	73	MFX	22.5	3	20	m
2	44	64	0.69	63	MFX	30.6	1	40	m
3	67	66	1.02	86	MFX	38.3	1.5	65	m
4	56	63	0.89	100	MFX	28.3	2	31	f
5	52	62	0.84	81	MFX	32.8	1	46	m
6	50	51	0.98	95	MFX	23.5	1	32	f
7	52	54	0.96	90	MFX	24.0	2	33	m
8	45	66	0.68	36	MFX	28.5	1.5	49	f
9	38	62	0.61	78	MFX	30.2	3.5	63	m
10	33	40	0.83	85	MFX	25.2	2.8	22	m
11	58	68	0.85	59	MFX	33.1	1	36	f
12	49	58	0.84	100	MFX	28.6	1.6	54	m
13	52	63	0.83	95	MFX	28.6	1.5	54	m
14	45	55	0.82	59	MFX	27.2	4	45	m
15	49	57	0.86	64	MFX	20.2	0.8	48	f
16	54	71	0.76	45	MFX	28.3	2	51	f
17	61	64	0.95	100	MFX	25.3	1	52	m
18	55	60	0.91	86	MFX	27.1	1.5	40	m
19	49	59	0.83	65	MFX	22.7	2	36	f
20	51	57	0.89	90	MFX	29.4	3	60	m
21	47	51	0.93	100	MFX	24.6	2.6	42	m
22	53	55	0.95	95	MFX	24.0	2.5	17	m
23	53	55	0.96	95	MFX	24.3	4.5	41	m
24	47	52	0.91	95	MFX	24.5	5	15	m

Table 2 – Part 1: Single case table relative T2 and clinical paramters – correlation analysis source data

25	42	50	0.84	91	Hyalograft	27.8	3	27	m
26	48	42	1.14	100	Hyalograft	23.7	4	29	m
27	43	43	1.01	92	Hyalograft	23.6	2.5	51	f
28	39	45	0.88	94	Hyalograft	22.0	7	39	m
29	49	48	1.01	76	Hyalograft	28.7	3	28	f
30	41	36	1.14	90	Hyalograft	19.1	1.5	21	f
31	19	29	0.65	82	Hyalograft	20.8	1.5	32	f
32	52	45	1.16	90	Hyalograft	19.6	6	19	m
33	46	42	1.10	94	Hyalograft	25.0	6	32	m
34	43	42	1.00	95	Hyalograft	29.3	4	25	m
35	40	48	0.84	85	BioCart II	23.2	3.1	38	m
36	46	43	1.07	90	BioCart II	20.6	3.1	30	m
37	45	46	0.98	75	BioCart II	21.3	7.1	27	m
38	42	49	0.85	85	BioCart II	24.3	7.1	40	m
39	65	63	1.04	90	BioCart II	25.5	4.9	31	m
40	63	60	1.06	90	BioCart II	25.5	7.1	32	m
Mean	47.9	53.3	0.91	83.8		25.80	3.08	37.3	
STD	8.92	9.67	0.13	15.34		4.05	1.91	12.82	
MIN	18	28	0.61	36		19.1	0.8	15	
MAX	67	71	1.16	100		38.3	7.1	65	

Table 2 – Part 2: Single case table of relative T2 and clinical paramters – correlation analysis source data

8 Figures

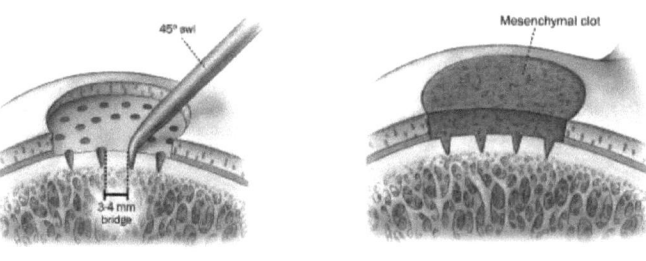

a b

Figure 1: Microfracture Technique [74]. After debridement of the chondral defect, microholes are set with a pick (a). Mechanical integrity of the subchondral plate has to be preserved. Subsequent bleeding introduces mesenchymal cells from the bone marrow that form a clot (b), which eventually forms repair tissue stabilizing the adjacent cartilage.

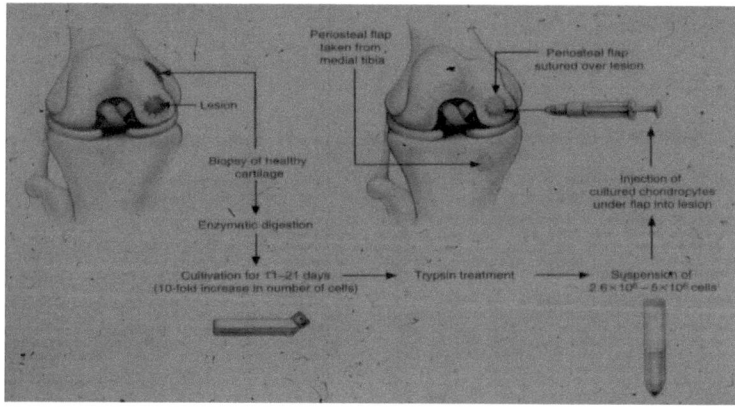

Figure 2: ACI with a periosteal flap as described by Peterson.

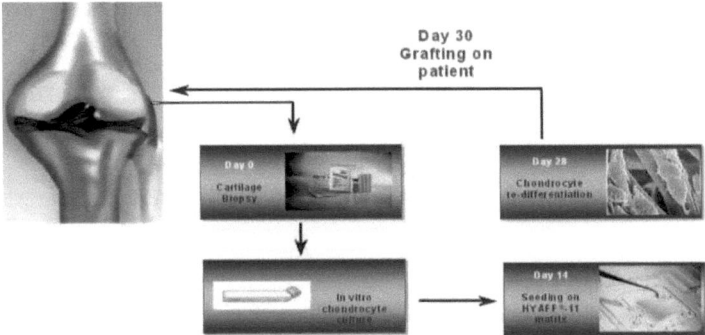

Figure 3: MACT with Hyalograft C.

Intrinsic	Extrinsic

• proton density
• T1 relaxation
• T1-ρ relaxation
• T2 relaxation
• cross relaxation
• dia- and ferromagnetic perturbations
• chemical shift
• temperature
• diffusion
• perfusion
• physiologic motion
• bulk flow
  (e.g., blood, CSF)
• viscosity
• changes of tissue composition
  (e.g., age, pathological changes)
	• static and gradient magnetic field strength
	• magnetic field homogeneity
	• hard- and software parameters
	  * type of coil
	  * number of slices, slice thickness and gaps, slice location and orientation
	  * number of averages
	  * pulse shape/bandwidth
	  * pixel and matrix size, field-of-view
	  * acquisition mode (2D/3D)
	  * artifact suppression
	  * triggering/gating
	  * orientation of phase- versus frequency-encoding gradients
	• RF pulse sequences and parameters
	• contrast-changing agents

Figure 4: Intrisic and extrinsic MRI parameters [74].

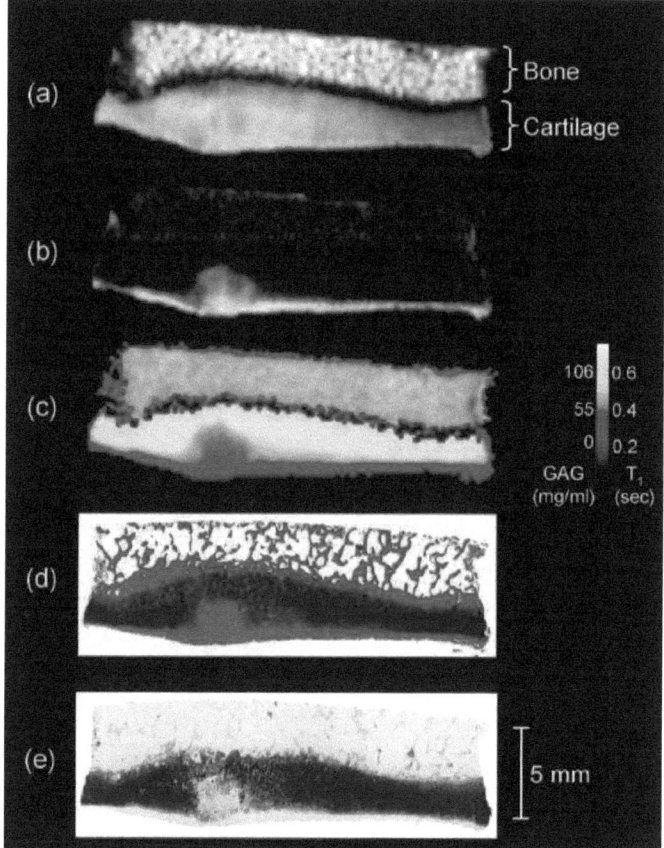

Figure 5: Comparison of morphological MRI, dGEMRIC and histology in a distinct cartilage sample [84].
(a) MRI image reflecting proton density, the cartilage appears intact.
(b) T1 weighted image post contrast; brighter areas indicate higher GdDTPA and hence lower GAG. An area of GAG depletion is obvious.
(c) Color coded T1 map with absolute T1 values (right side of the color bar), reflecting GAG (left side of the color bar).
(d) HE staining validates that the cartilage is intact, the pattern of staining corresponds with the MRI image
(e) Toluidine blue staining verifies the absence of GAG in the area delineated by post contrast T1 imaging

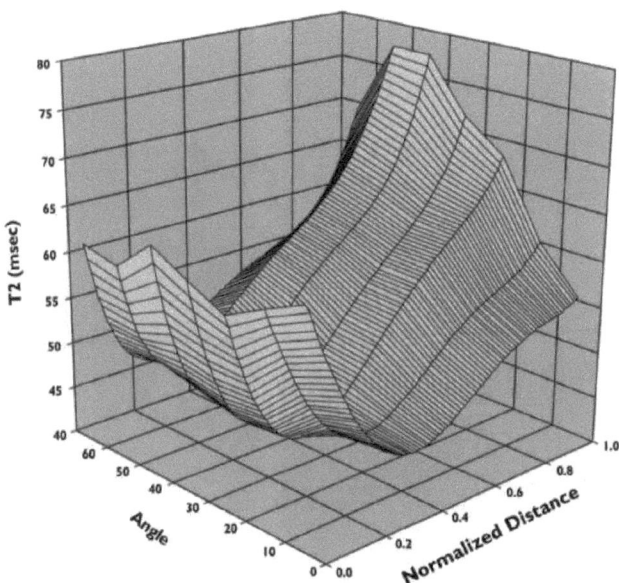

Figure 6: Zonal variation of T2 in cartilage under consideration of the magic angle defect at 3T in vivo [160]. Superficial layers are more prone to the magic angle effect, however a reliable assessment of the cartilage layers is possible.

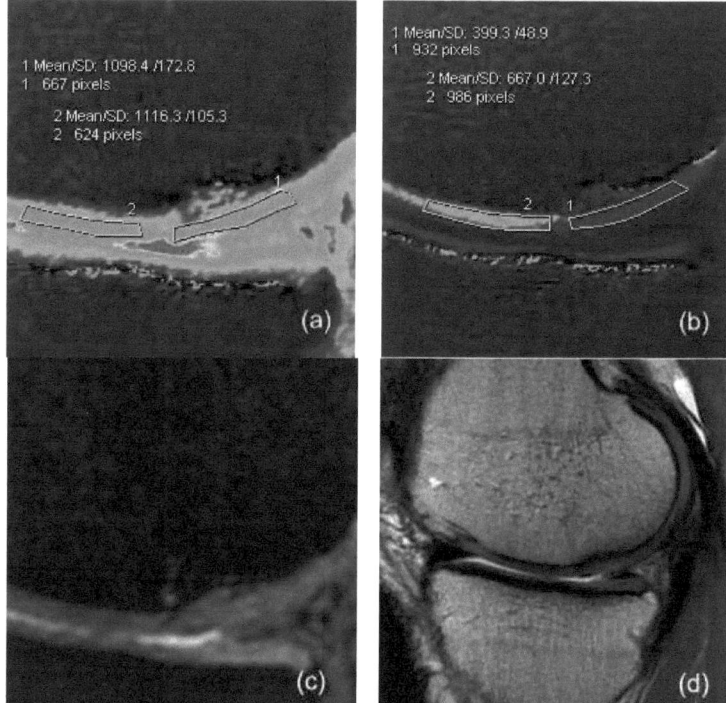

Figure 7 [140]: Example of the evaluation of T1 and T2 maps (patient after autologous chondrocyte implantation with a fibrin scaffold). The regions of interest (ROI) are defined under consideration of high resolution morphologic MR images (7c, DESS Sequence, and 7d, proton desity weighted image). Subsequently ROIs are placed pre contrast T1 (a) and post contrast T1 (b) analysis. ROIs have to be placed in the same locations pre and post contrast to evaluate the relative delta relaxation rate (rΔR1). ROIs can be copied from pre to post contrast maps (c) in order to ensure the exact evaluation of rΔR1. Mark the difference of the RT area (ROI #1 a/b) and the RC area (ROI #2 a/b) pre- and post-contrast.

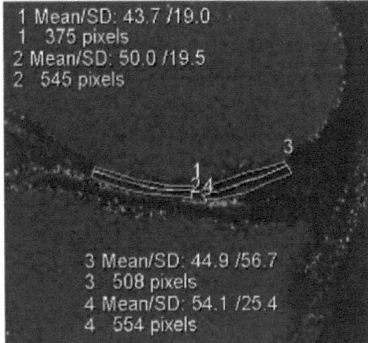 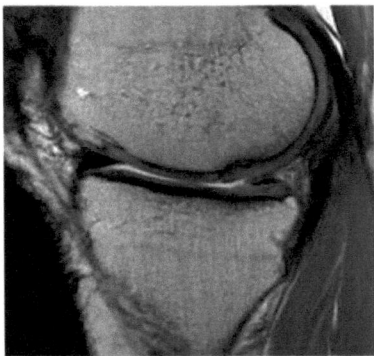

Figure: T2-map region of interest (ROI) evaluation with the corresponding morphological image of the case shown in Figure 7. ROI #1: deep reference cartilage (RC), ROI #2: superficial RC, ROI #3 : deep repair tissue (RT), ROI #4: superficial RT. Both RC and RT show a marked increase towards the surface in this case.

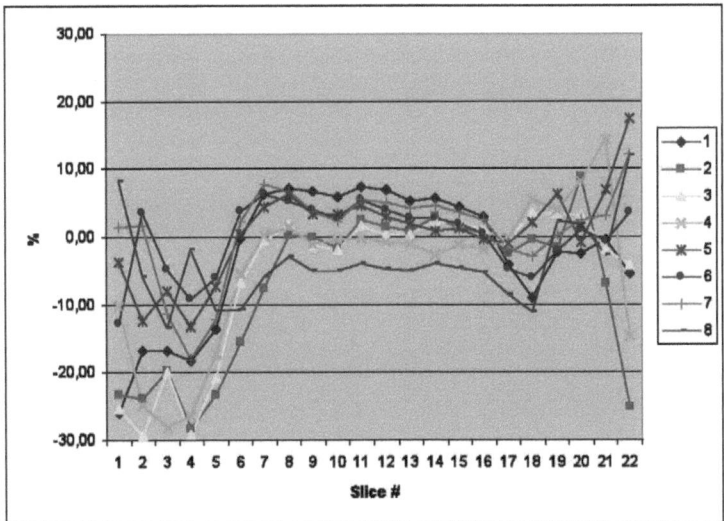

Figure 8: Differences of T1 between the IR and the VIBE sequence in the 8 phantoms expressed as % of IR over the slab profile. The central slices show acceptable agreement, however, the values in the peripheral 5 slices cannot be considered sufficiently accurate. There is a tendency towards slightly higher T1 in the VIBE sequence.

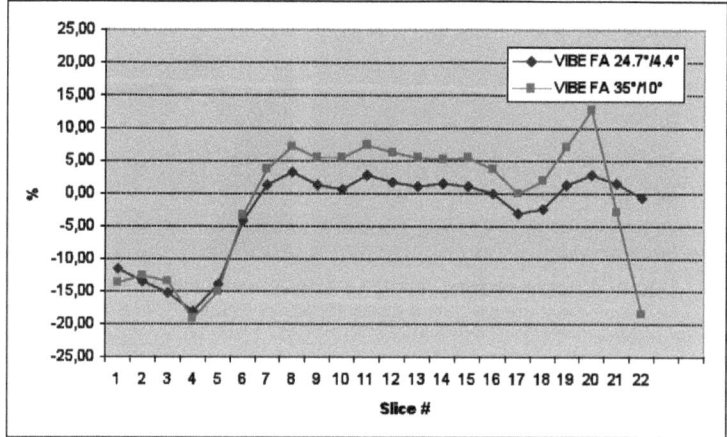

Figure 9: The central slices (6-17) have considerable better accuracy due to the RF homogeneity profile than the slices at the periphery (1-5, 17-22). The y-axis gives the difference between T1 measured by the inversion recovery sequence and by the 3D dual flip angle techniques in percent (%).

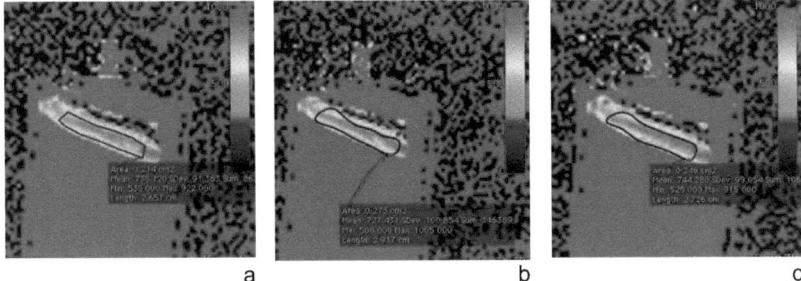

Figure 10: ROI settings in the repeated measurements in cartilage sample C (a-c).

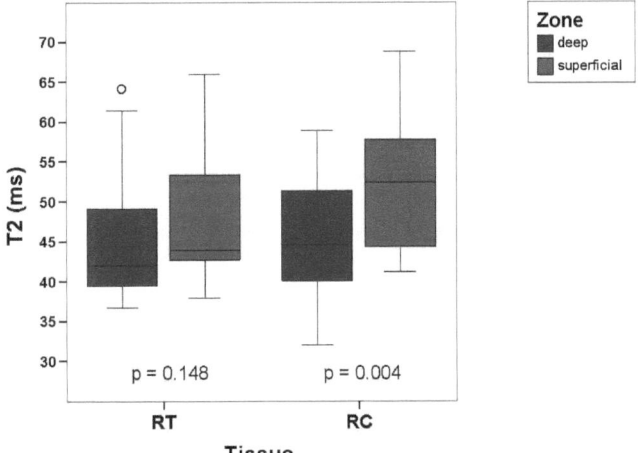

Figure 11: Bi-laminar evaluation: mean values of T2 in normal, hyaline reference cartilage (RC) and cartilage repair tissue (RT) in the deep and superficial zones after Biocart II™.

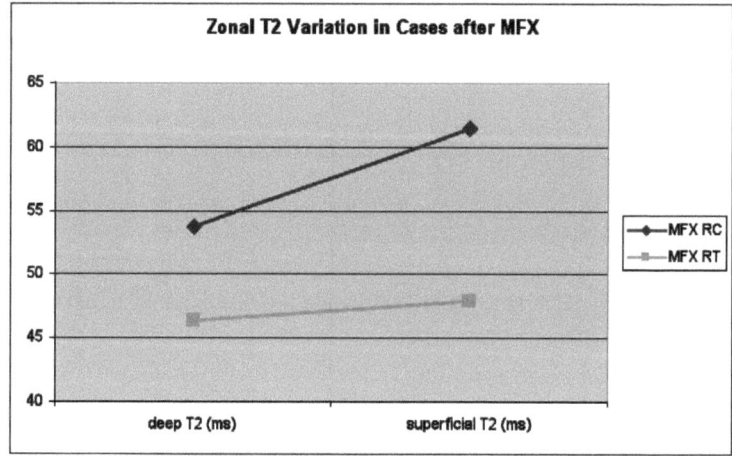
(a)

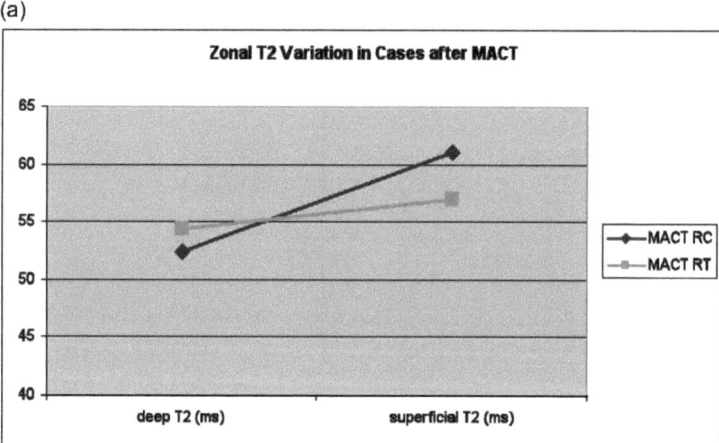
(b)
Figure 12: Zonal variation of T2 in normal reference cartilage and in repair tissue after MFX (a) and MACT (b) assessed in bi-laminar region of interest analysis. The T2 values differ significantly between deep and superficial reference cartilage (RC) both in the cases after MFX and MACT. In contrast, there is a significant difference only in the repair tissue (RT) after MACT, but not after MFX.

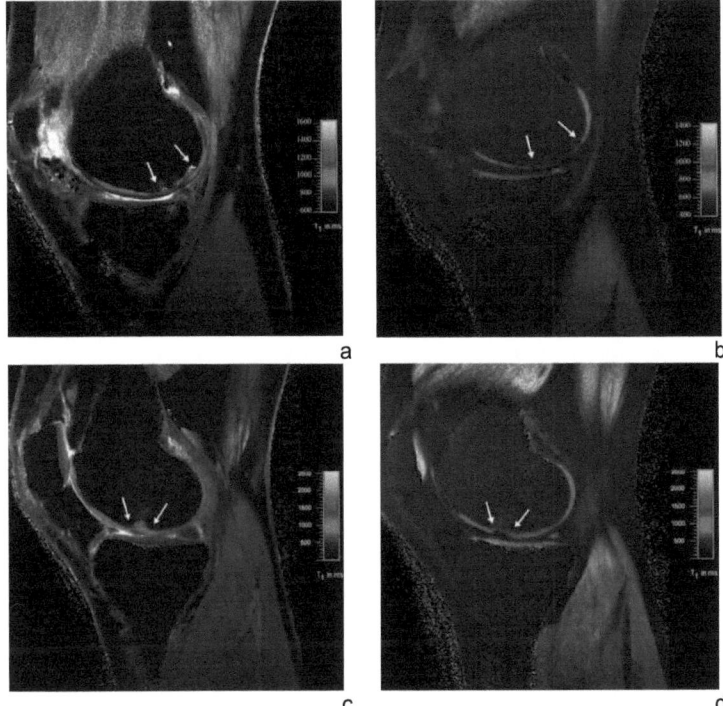

Figure 13: MACT (Hyalograft, a, b) and MFX (c,d) pre- and post-contrast T1 maps [162]. Both MACT and MFX tissue show decreased T1 in comparison to adjacent cartilage.

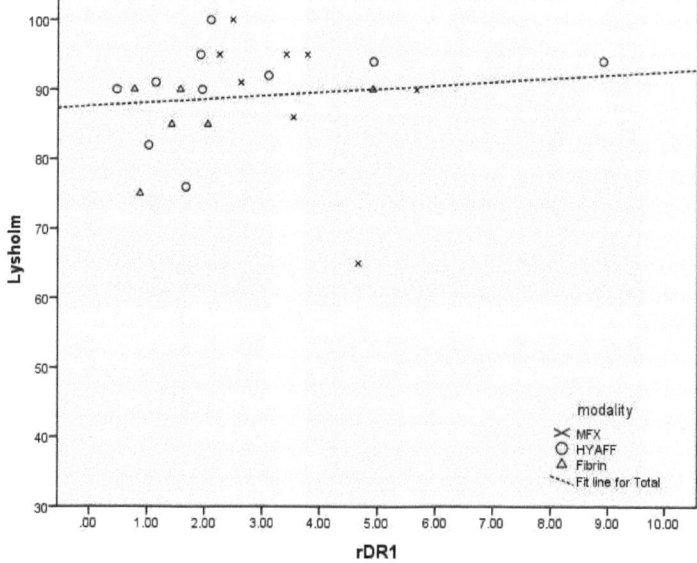

Figure 14: Correlation of the relative delta relaxation rate (rΔR1) and the Lysholm Score in 24 cartilage repair patients after different procedures (MFX – Microfracture, HYAFF – Hyalograft, Fibrin – BioCart II). Obviously clinical outcome is not related to repair tissue fixed charge density assessed with rΔR1.

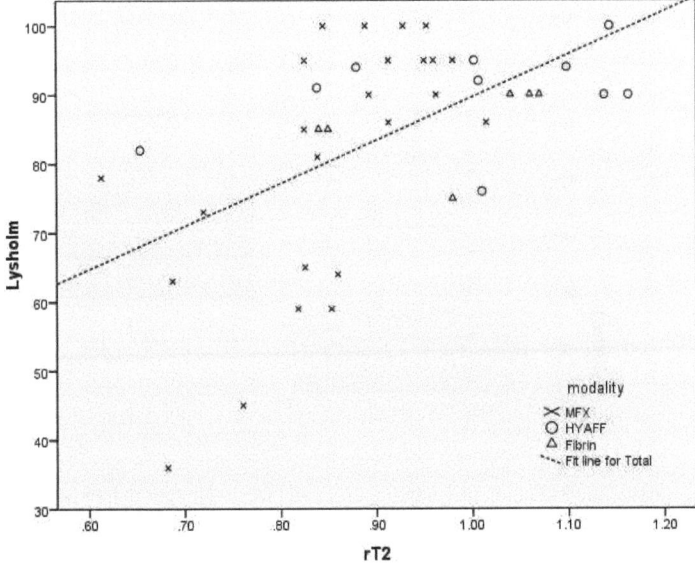

Figure 15: Scatterplot of rT2 and the Lysholm Score after different cartilage repair procedures (MFX – Microfracture, HYAFF – Hyalograft, Fibrin – BioCart II) with linear regression. A moderate but significant correlation (Spearman's rho r_s = 0.491, p = 0.001) is found, and multiple linear regression analysis yields a moderate predictive value of rT2 for the Lysholm Score (R^2 = 0.298) under consideration of age and treatment modality as confounding variables.

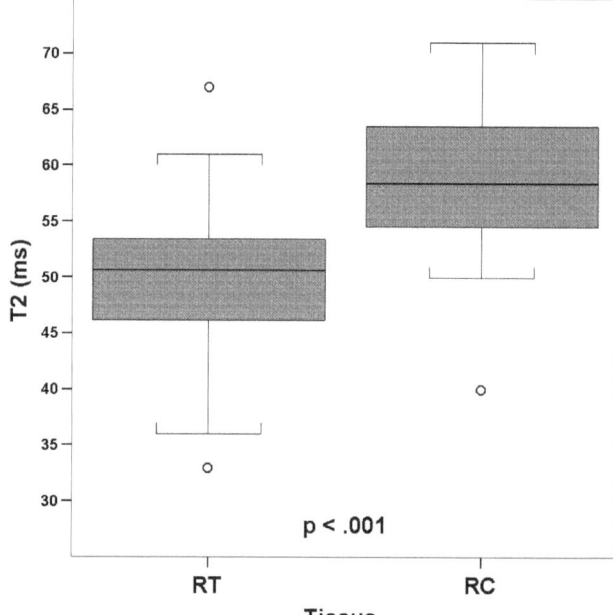

Figure 16: Boxplot of the T2 values in microfracture repair tissue (RT) and in articular reference cartilage (RC). RT T2 values differ significantly from RC T2 in the paired student t-test (N = 24).

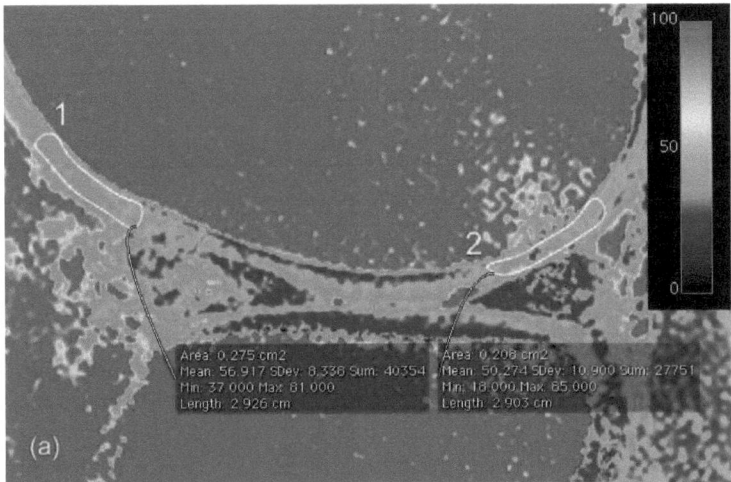

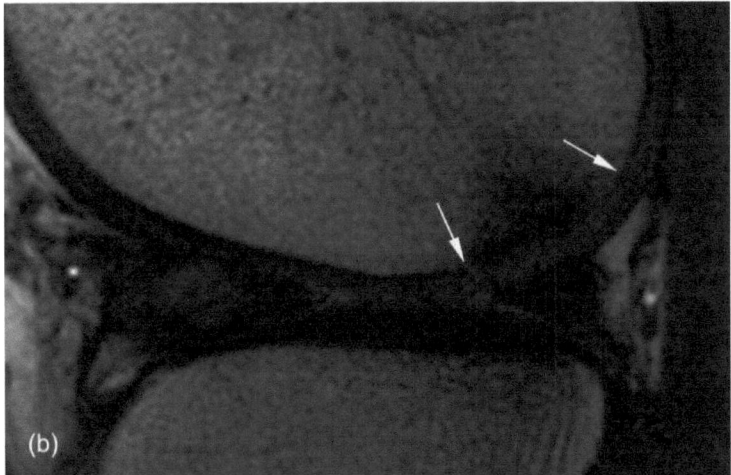

Figure17: Example of global T2 assessment in a case after MFX. This case had 95 points in the Lysholm Score at the time of the MR examination. The T2 map (a) is evaluated in consensus with the morphological image (b) where the repair site is clearly delineated by the structure alteration of the subchondral bone subsequent to the MFX treatment (white arrows). The reference cartilage (1, 56.9 ms) should be

chosen so that it has a comparable orientation to B1 like the repair site (2, 50.3 ms). The regions of interest should cover the full thickness of the cartilage layer, but must not include subchondral bone or joint fluid.

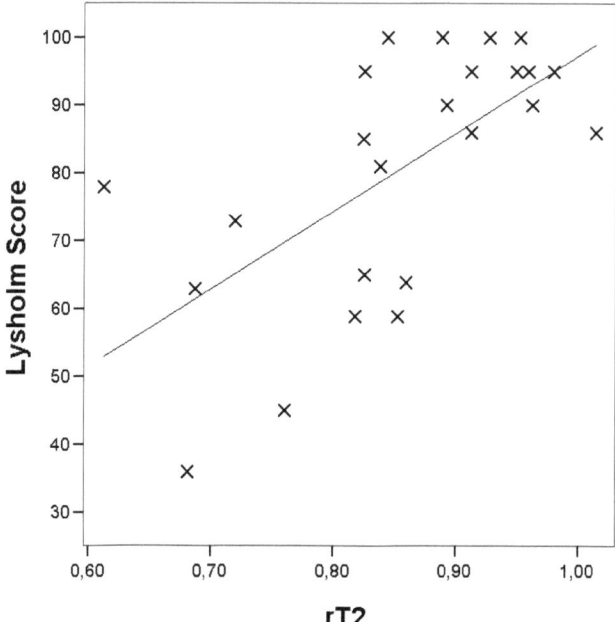

Figure 18: Scatterplot with linear fitting indicating the rank correlation (Spearman's rho: $r_s = 0.641$, $p < 0.001$) of relative T2 (rT2) with the Lysholm Score

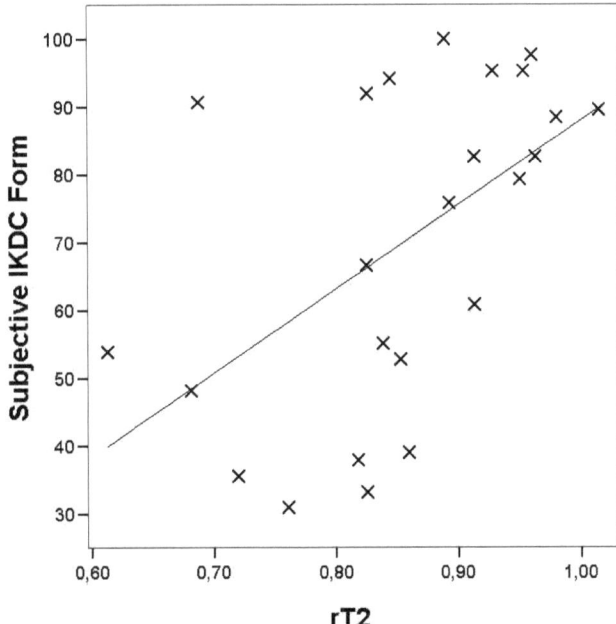

Figure 19: Scatterplot with linear fitting indicating the rank correlation (Spearman´s rho: r_s = 0.549, p = 0.005) of relative T2 (rT2) with the Subjective IKDC Form.

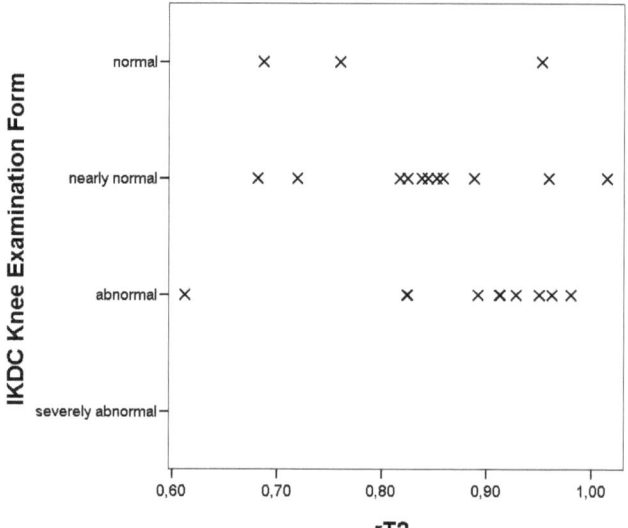

Figure 20: Scatterplot of relative T2 (rT2) with the IKDC Knee Examination Form. Spearman's rho analysis does not indicate a relationship between the variables (r_s = -0.284, p = 0.179).

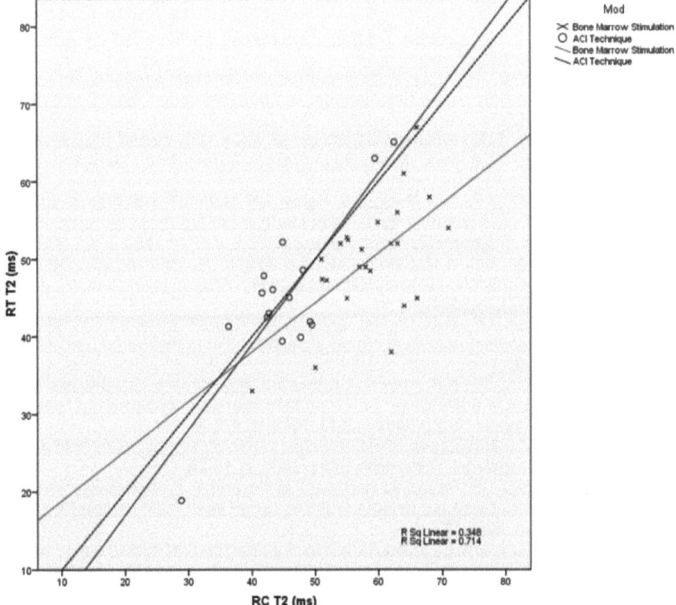

Figure 21: Linear regression fit analyses comparing RT T2 and RC T2 in MFX and in MACT. The black line symbolizes perfect outcome, meaning that RT T2 = RC T2. The analyses suggest the cases after MACT have better outcome, as the fit is close to RT = RC T2 and R2 is higher than after MFX indicating that cartilage repair with MACT is more likely to result in repair tissue with T2 comparable to the native articular cartilage.

9 References

1. Nehrer, S. and T. Minas, *Treatment of articular cartilage defects. Invest Radiol, 2000. 35(10): p. 639-46.*
2. Buckwalter, J.A. and H.J. Mankin, *Articular cartilage: degeneration and osteoarthritis, repair, regeneration, and transplantation. Instr Course Lect, 1998. 47: p. 487-504.*
3. Hunziker, E.B., *Articular cartilage repair: basic science and clinical progress. A review of the current status and prospects. Osteoarthritis Cartilage, 2002. 10(6): p. 432-63.*
4. Steadman, J.R., B.S. Miller, S.G. Karas, T.F. Schlegel, K.K. Briggs, and R.J. Hawkins, *The microfracture technique in the treatment of full-thickness chondral lesions of the knee in National Football League players. J Knee Surg, 2003. 16(2): p. 83-6.*
5. Steadman, J.R., W.G. Rodkey, and K.K. Briggs, *Microfracture to treat full-thickness chondral defects: surgical technique, rehabilitation, and outcomes. J Knee Surg, 2002. 15(3): p. 170-6.*
6. Steadman, J.R., W.G. Rodkey, and J.J. Rodrigo, *Microfracture: surgical technique and rehabilitation to treat chondral defects. Clin Orthop Relat Res, 2001(391 Suppl): p. S362-9.*
7. Steadman, J.R., K.K. Briggs, J.J. Rodrigo, M.S. Kocher, T.J. Gill, and W.G. Rodkey, *Outcomes of microfracture for traumatic chondral defects of the knee: average 11-year follow-up. Arthroscopy, 2003. 19(5): p. 477-84.*
8. Bobic, V., *[Autologous osteo-chondral grafts in the management of articular cartilage lesions]. Orthopade, 1999. 28(1): p. 19-25.*
9. Hangody, L., P. Feczko, L. Bartha, G. Bodo, and G. Kish, *Mosaicplasty for the treatment of articular defects of the knee and ankle. Clin Orthop Relat Res, 2001(391 Suppl): p. S328-36.*
10. Hangody, L. and P. Fules, *Autologous osteochondral mosaicplasty for the treatment of full-thickness defects of weight-bearing joints: ten years of experimental and clinical experience. J Bone Joint Surg Am, 2003. 85-A Suppl 2: p. 25-32.*
11. Hangody, L., G.K. Rathonyi, Z. Duska, G. Vasarhelyi, P. Fules, and L. Modis, *Autologous osteochondral mosaicplasty. Surgical technique. J Bone Joint Surg Am, 2004. 86-A Suppl 1: p. 65-72.*
12. Brittberg, M., *Autologous chondrocyte transplantation. Clin Orthop Relat Res, 1999(367 Suppl): p. S147-55.*
13. Brittberg, M., A. Lindahl, A. Nilsson, C. Ohlsson, O. Isaksson, and L. Peterson, *Treatment of deep cartilage defects in the knee with autologous chondrocyte transplantation. N Engl J Med, 1994. 331(14): p. 889-95.*
14. Peterson, L., M. Brittberg, I. Kiviranta, E.L. Akerlund, and A. Lindahl, *Autologous chondrocyte transplantation. Biomechanics and long-term durability. Am J Sports Med, 2002. 30(1): p. 2-12.*
15. Peterson, L., T. Minas, M. Brittberg, A. Nilsson, E. Sjogren-Jansson, and A. Lindahl, *Two- to 9-year outcome after autologous chondrocyte transplantation of the knee. Clin Orthop Relat Res, 2000(374): p. 212-34.*
16. Knutsen, G., L. Engebretsen, T.C. Ludvigsen, J.O. Drogset, T. Grontvedt, E. Solheim, et al., *Autologous chondrocyte implantation compared with microfracture in the knee. A randomized trial. J Bone Joint Surg Am, 2004. 86-A(3): p. 455-64.*
17. Mithoefer, K., R.J. Williams, 3rd, R.F. Warren, H.G. Potter, C.R. Spock, E.C. Jones, et al., *The microfracture technique for the treatment of articular cartilage lesions in the knee. A prospective cohort study. J Bone Joint Surg Am, 2005. 87(9): p. 1911-20.*
18. Szerb, I., L. Hangody, Z. Duska, and N.P. Kaposi, *Mosaicplasty: long-term follow-up. Bull Hosp Jt Dis, 2005. 63(1-2): p. 54-62.*
19. Henderson, I., B. Tuy, and B. Oakes, *Reoperation after autologous chondrocyte implantation. Indications and findings. J Bone Joint Surg Br, 2004. 86(2): p. 205-11.*
20. Nehrer, S., H.A. Breinan, A. Ramappa, G. Young, S. Shortkroff, L.K. Louie, et al., *Matrix collagen type and pore size influence behaviour of seeded canine chondrocytes. Biomaterials, 1997. 18(11): p. 769-76.*

21. *Nehrer, S., H.A. Breinan, A. Ramappa, S. Shortkroff, G. Young, T. Minas, et al., Canine chondrocytes seeded in type I and type II collagen implants investigated in vitro. J Biomed Mater Res, 1997. 38(2): p. 95-104.*
22. *Dorotka, R., U. Windberger, K. Macfelda, U. Bindreiter, C. Toma, and S. Nehrer, Repair of articular cartilage defects treated by microfracture and a three-dimensional collagen matrix. Biomaterials, 2005. 26(17): p. 3617-29.*
23. *Dorotka, R., U. Bindreiter, K. Macfelda, U. Windberger, and S. Nehrer, Marrow stimulation and chondrocyte transplantation using a collagen matrix for cartilage repair. Osteoarthritis Cartilage, 2005. 13(8): p. 655-64.*
24. *Nehrer, S., S. Domayer, R. Dorotka, K. Schatz, U. Bindreiter, and R. Kotz, Three-year clinical outcome after chondrocyte transplantation using a hyaluronan matrix for cartilage repair. Eur J Radiol, 2006. 57(1): p. 3-8.*
25. *Marcacci, M., M. Berruto, D. Brocchetta, A. Delcogliano, D. Ghinelli, A. Gobbi, et al., Articular cartilage engineering with Hyalograft C: 3-year clinical results. Clin Orthop Relat Res, 2005(435): p. 96-105.*
26. *Marcacci, M., S. Zaffagnini, E. Kon, A. Visani, F. Iacono, and I. Loreti, Arthroscopic autologous chondrocyte transplantation: technical note. Knee Surg Sports Traumatol Arthrosc, 2002. 10(3): p. 154-9.*
27. *Sittinger, M., D. Reitzel, M. Dauner, H. Hierlemann, C. Hammer, E. Kastenbauer, et al., Resorbable polyesters in cartilage engineering: affinity and biocompatibility of polymer fiber structures to chondrocytes. J Biomed Mater Res, 1996. 33(2): p. 57-63.*
28. *Chu, C.R., R.D. Coutts, M. Yoshioka, F.L. Harwood, A.Z. Monosov, and D. Amiel, Articular cartilage repair using allogeneic perichondrocyte-seeded biodegradable porous polylactic acid (PLA): a tissue-engineering study. J Biomed Mater Res, 1995. 29(9): p. 1147-54.*
29. *Grigolo, B., G. Lisignoli, A. Piacentini, M. Fiorini, P. Gobbi, G. Mazzotti, et al., Evidence for redifferentiation of human chondrocytes grown on a hyaluronan-based biomaterial (HYAff 11): molecular, immunohistochemical and ultrastructural analysis. Biomaterials, 2002. 23(4): p. 1187-95.*
30. *Behrens, P., T. Bitter, B. Kurz, and M. Russlies, Matrix-associated autologous chondrocyte transplantation/implantation (MACT/MACI)--5-year follow-up. Knee, 2006. 13(3): p. 194-202.*
31. *Bartlett, W., C.R. Gooding, R.W. Carrington, J.A. Skinner, T.W. Briggs, and G. Bentley, Autologous chondrocyte implantation at the knee using a bilayer collagen membrane with bone graft. A preliminary report. J Bone Joint Surg Br, 2005. 87(3): p. 330-2.*
32. *Bartlett W, S.J., Gooding CR, Carrington RW, Flanagan AM, Briggs TW, and B. G., Autologous chondrocyte implantation versus matrix-induced autologous chondrocyte implantation for osteochondral defects of the knee: a prospective, randomised study. J Bone Joint Surg Br., 2005 May. 87(5): p. 640-5.*
33. *Smith, G.D., G. Knutsen, and J.B. Richardson, A clinical review of cartilage repair techniques. J Bone Joint Surg Br, 2005. 87(4): p. 445-9.*
34. *Kish, G., L. Modis, and L. Hangody, Osteochondral mosaicplasty for the treatment of focal chondral and osteochondral lesions of the knee and talus in the athlete. Rationale, indications, techniques, and results. Clin Sports Med, 1999. 18(1): p. 45-66, vi.*
35. *Jakob, R.P., T. Franz, E. Gautier, and P. Mainil-Varlet, Autologous osteochondral grafting in the knee: indication, results, and reflections. Clin Orthop Relat Res, 2002(401): p. 170-84.*
36. *Kreuz, P.C., C. Erggelet, M.R. Steinwachs, S.J. Krause, A. Lahm, P. Niemeyer, et al., Is microfracture of chondral defects in the knee associated with different results in patients aged 40 years or younger? Arthroscopy, 2006. 22(11): p. 1180-6.*
37. *Kreuz, P.C., M.R. Steinwachs, C. Erggelet, S.J. Krause, G. Konrad, M. Uhl, et al., Results after microfracture of full-thickness chondral defects in different compartments in the knee. Osteoarthritis Cartilage, 2006. 14(11): p. 1119-25.*
38. *Gobbi, A., P. Nunag, and K. Malinowski, Treatment of full thickness chondral lesions of the knee with microfracture in a group of athletes. Knee Surg Sports Traumatol Arthrosc, 2005. 13(3): p. 213-21.*

39. *Brittberg, M. and C.S. Winalski, Evaluation of cartilage injuries and repair. J Bone Joint Surg Am, 2003. 85-A Suppl 2: p. 58-69.*
40. *Micheli, L.J., J.E. Browne, C. Erggelet, F. Fu, B. Mandelbaum, J.B. Moseley, et al., Autologous chondrocyte implantation of the knee: multicenter experience and minimum 3-year follow-up. Clin J Sport Med, 2001. 11(4): p. 223-8.*
41. *Peterson, L., T. Minas, M. Brittberg, and A. Lindahl, Treatment of osteochondritis dissecans of the knee with autologous chondrocyte transplantation: results at two to ten years. J Bone Joint Surg Am, 2003. 85-A Suppl 2: p. 17-24.*
42. *Henderson, I., P. Lavigne, H. Valenzuela, and B. Oakes, Autologous chondrocyte implantation: superior biologic properties of hyaline cartilage repairs. Clin Orthop Relat Res, 2007. 455: p. 253-61.*
43. *Henderson IJ, T.B., Connell D, Oakes B, Hettwer WH., Prospective clinical study of autologous chondrocyte implantation and correlation with MRI at three and 12 months. J Bone Joint Surg Br., 2003. Sep;85((7)): p. 1060-6.*
44. *Watanabe, A., Y. Wada, T. Obata, T. Sasho, T. Ueda, M. Tamura, et al., Time course evaluation of reparative cartilage with MR imaging after autologous chondrocyte implantation. Cell Transplant, 2005. 14(9): p. 695-700.*
45. *Tins, B.J., I.W. McCall, T. Takahashi, V. Cassar-Pullicino, S. Roberts, B. Ashton, et al., Autologous chondrocyte implantation in knee joint: MR imaging and histologic features at 1-year follow-up. Radiology, 2005. 234(2): p. 501-8.*
46. *Marlovits, S., P. Zeller, P. Singer, C. Resinger, and V. Vecsei, Cartilage repair: generations of autologous chondrocyte transplantation. Eur J Radiol, 2006. 57(1): p. 24-31.*
47. *Pavesio, A., G. Abatangelo, A. Borrione, D. Brocchetta, A.P. Hollander, E. Kon, et al., Hyaluronan-based scaffolds (Hyalograft C) in the treatment of knee cartilage defects: preliminary clinical findings. Novartis Found Symp, 2003. 249: p. 203-17; discussion 229-33, 234-8, 239-41.*
48. *Knutsen, G., J.O. Drogset, L. Engebretsen, T. Grontvedt, V. Isaksen, T.C. Ludvigsen, et al., A randomized trial comparing autologous chondrocyte implantation with microfracture. Findings at five years. J Bone Joint Surg Am, 2007. 89(10): p. 2105-12.*
49. *Wasiak J, C.C., Villanueva E., Autologous cartilage implantation for full thickness articular cartilage defects of the knee. Cochrane Database Syst, 2006. Jul 19;3:CD003323 Review.*
50. *Bentley, G., L.C. Biant, R.W. Carrington, M. Akmal, A. Goldberg, A.M. Williams, et al., A prospective, randomised comparison of autologous chondrocyte implantation versus mosaicplasty for osteochondral defects in the knee. J Bone Joint Surg Br, 2003. 85(2): p. 223-30.*
51. *Saris, D.B., J. Vanlauwe, J. Victor, M. Haspl, M. Bohnsack, Y. Fortems, et al., Characterized chondrocyte implantation results in better structural repair when treating symptomatic cartilage defects of the knee in a randomized controlled trial versus microfracture. Am J Sports Med, 2008. 36(2): p. 235-46.*
52. *Gooding CR, B.W., Bentley G, Skinner JA, Carrington R, Flanagan A, A prospective, ranomised study comparing two techniques of autologous chondrocyte implantation for osteochondral defects in the knee: Periosteum covered versus type I/III collagen covered. The Knee, 2006. 13: p. 203-210.*
53. *Gobbi, A., E. Kon, M. Berruto, R. Francisco, G. Filardo, and M. Marcacci, Patellofemoral full-thickness chondral defects treated with Hyalograft-C: a clinical, arthroscopic, and histologic review. Am J Sports Med, 2006. 34(11): p. 1763-73.*
54. *Kon, E., A. Gobbi, G. Filardo, M. Delcogliano, S. Zaffagnini, and M. Marcacci, Arthroscopic second-generation autologous chondrocyte implantation compared with microfracture for chondral lesions of the knee: prospective nonrandomized study at 5 years. Am J Sports Med, 2009. 37(1): p. 33-41.*
55. *van den Borne, M.P., N.J. Raijmakers, J. Vanlauwe, J. Victor, S.N. de Jong, J. Bellemans, et al., International Cartilage Repair Society (ICRS) and Oswestry macroscopic cartilage evaluation scores validated for use in Autologous Chondrocyte Implantation (ACI) and microfracture. Osteoarthritis Cartilage, 2007. 15(12): p. 1397-402.*
56. *Nehrer, S., M. Spector, and T. Minas, Histologic analysis of tissue after failed cartilage repair procedures. Clin Orthop Relat Res, 1999(365): p. 149-62.*

57. Roberts S, M.I., Darby AJ, Menage J, Evans H, Harrison PE, Richardson JB., Autologous chondrocyte implantation for cartilage repair: monitoring its success by magnetic resonance imaging and histology. Arthritis Res Ther., 2003. 5:((1)): p. R60-73.
58. Moriya, T., Y. Wada, A. Watanabe, T. Sasho, K. Nakagawa, P. Mainil-Varlet, et al., Evaluation of reparative cartilage after autologous chondrocyte implantation for osteochondritis dissecans: histology, biochemistry, and MR imaging. J Orthop Sci, 2007. 12(3): p. 265-73.
59. Trattnig, S., Overuse of hyaline cartilage and imaging. Eur J Radiol, 1997. 25(3): p. 188-98.
60. Recht, M., V. Bobic, D. Burstein, D. Disler, G. Gold, M. Gray, et al., Magnetic resonance imaging of articular cartilage. Clin Orthop Relat Res, 2001(391 Suppl): p. S379-96.
61. Disler, D.G., T.R. McCauley, C.G. Kelman, M.D. Fuchs, L.M. Ratner, C.R. Wirth, et al., Fat-suppressed three-dimensional spoiled gradient-echo MR imaging of hyaline cartilage defects in the knee: comparison with standard MR imaging and arthroscopy. AJR Am J Roentgenol, 1996. 167(1): p. 127-32.
62. Potter, H.G., J.M. Linklater, A.A. Allen, J.A. Hannafin, and S.B. Haas, Magnetic resonance imaging of articular cartilage in the knee. An evaluation with use of fast-spin-echo imaging. J Bone Joint Surg Am, 1998. 80(9): p. 1276-84.
63. Bobic, V., ICRS articular cartilage imaging committee, ICRS MR Imaging Protocol for knee articular cartilage. Newsletter 2000, III, 2000: p. 12.
64. Yao, L., A. Gentili, and A. Thomas, Incidental magnetization transfer contrast in fast spin-echo imaging of cartilage. J Magn Reson Imaging, 1996. 6(1): p. 180-4.
65. Constable, R.T., A.W. Anderson, J. Zhong, and J.C. Gore, Factors influencing contrast in fast spin-echo MR imaging. Magn Reson Imaging, 1992. 10(4): p. 497-511.
66. Burkart, A. and A.B. Imhoff, [Diagnostic imaging after autologous chondrocyte transplantation. Correlation of magnetic resonance tomography, histological and arthroscopic findings]. Orthopade, 2000. 29(2): p. 135-44.
67. Trattnig, S., M. Huber, M.J. Breitenseher, H.J. Trnka, T. Rand, A. Kaider, et al., Imaging articular cartilage defects with 3D fat-suppressed echo planar imaging: comparison with conventional 3D fat-suppressed gradient echo sequence and correlation with histology. J Comput Assist Tomogr, 1998. 22(1): p. 8-14.
68. Duc, S.R., C.W. Pfirrmann, M.R. Schmid, M. Zanetti, P.P. Koch, F. Kalberer, et al., Articular cartilage defects detected with 3D water-excitation true FISP: prospective comparison with sequences commonly used for knee imaging. Radiology, 2007. 245(1): p. 216-23.
69. Eckstein, F., M. Hudelmaier, W. Wirth, B. Kiefer, R. Jackson, J. Yu, et al., Double echo steady state magnetic resonance imaging of knee articular cartilage at 3 Tesla: a pilot study for the Osteoarthritis Initiative. Ann Rheum Dis, 2006. 65(4): p. 433-41.
70. Welsch, G.H., T.C. Mamisch, T. Hughes, S. Domayer, S. Marlovits, and S. Trattnig, Advanced morphological and biochemical magnetic resonance imaging of cartilage repair procedures in the knee joint at 3 Tesla. Semin Musculoskelet Radiol, 2008. 12(3): p. 196-211.
71. Peterfy, C.G., C.F. van Dijke, Y. Lu, A. Nguyen, T.J. Connick, J.B. Kneeland, et al., Quantification of the volume of articular cartilage in the metacarpophalangeal joints of the hand: accuracy and precision of three-dimensional MR imaging. AJR Am J Roentgenol, 1995. 165(2): p. 371-5.
72. Recht, M.P., D.W. Piraino, G.A. Paletta, J.P. Schils, and G.H. Belhobek, Accuracy of fat-suppressed three-dimensional spoiled gradient-echo FLASH MR imaging in the detection of patellofemoral articular cartilage abnormalities. Radiology, 1996. 198(1): p. 209-12.
73. Rubenstein, J.D., J.G. Li, S. Majumdar, and R.M. Henkelman, Image resolution and signal-to-noise ratio requirements for MR imaging of degenerative cartilage. AJR Am J Roentgenol, 1997. 169(4): p. 1089-96.
74. Rinck, P.A., Magnetic Resonance in Medicine: The Basic Textbook of the European Magnetic Resonance Forum. 5th editition. ISBN 3-936072-12-4, 2003.

75. *Maroudas, A., H. Muir, and J. Wingham, The correlation of fixed negative charge with glycosaminoglycan content of human articular cartilage. Biochim Biophys Acta, 1969. 177(3): p. 492-500.*
76. *Bashir, A., M.L. Gray, R.D. Boutin, and D. Burstein, Glycosaminoglycan in articular cartilage: in vivo assessment with delayed Gd(DTPA)(2-)-enhanced MR imaging. Radiology, 1997. 205(2): p. 551-8.*
77. *Bashir, A., M.L. Gray, and D. Burstein, Gd-DTPA2- as a measure of cartilage degradation. Magn Reson Med, 1996. 36(5): p. 665-73.*
78. *Bashir, A., M.L. Gray, J. Hartke, and D. Burstein, Nondestructive imaging of human cartilage glycosaminoglycan concentration by MRI. Magn Reson Med, 1999. 41(5): p. 857-65.*
79. *Nieminen, M.T., J. Rieppo, J. Silvennoinen, J. Toyras, J.M. Hakumaki, M.M. Hyttinen, et al., Spatial assessment of articular cartilage proteoglycans with Gd-DTPA-enhanced T1 imaging. Magn Reson Med, 2002. 48(4): p. 640-8.*
80. *Burstein, D., J. Velyvis, K.T. Scott, K.W. Stock, Y.J. Kim, D. Jaramillo, et al., Protocol issues for delayed Gd(DTPA)(2-)-enhanced MRI (dGEMRIC) for clinical evaluation of articular cartilage. Magn Reson Med, 2001. 45(1): p. 36-41.*
81. *Burstein, D. and M.L. Gray, Is MRI fulfilling its promise for molecular imaging of cartilage in arthritis? Osteoarthritis Cartilage, 2006. 14(11): p. 1087-90.*
82. *Nieminen, M.T., J. Rieppo, J. Toyras, J.M. Hakumaki, J. Silvennoinen, M.M. Hyttinen, et al., T2 relaxation reveals spatial collagen architecture in articular cartilage: a comparative quantitative MRI and polarized light microscopic study. Magn Reson Med, 2001. 46(3): p. 487-93.*
83. *Grunder, W., M. Wagner, and A. Werner, MR-microscopic visualization of anisotropic internal cartilage structures using the magic angle technique. Magn Reson Med, 1998. 39(3): p. 376-82.*
84. *Mosher, T.J., H. Smith, B.J. Dardzinski, V.J. Schmithorst, and M.B. Smith, MR imaging and T2 mapping of femoral cartilage: in vivo determination of the magic angle effect. AJR Am J Roentgenol, 2001. 177(3): p. 665-9.*
85. *Wayne, J.S., K.A. Kraft, K.J. Shields, C. Yin, J.R. Owen, and D.G. Disler, MR imaging of normal and matrix-depleted cartilage: correlation with biomechanical function and biochemical composition. Radiology, 2003. 228(2): p. 493-9.*
86. *Li, X., C. Benjamin Ma, T.M. Link, D.D. Castillo, G. Blumenkrantz, J. Lozano, et al., In vivo T(1rho) and T(2) mapping of articular cartilage in osteoarthritis of the knee using 3 T MRI. Osteoarthritis Cartilage, 2007. 15(7): p. 789-97.*
87. *Alparslan, L., T. Minas, and C.S. Winalski, Magnetic resonance imaging of autologous chondrocyte implantation. Semin Ultrasound CT MR, 2001. 22(4): p. 341-51.*
88. *Alparslan, L., C.S. Winalski, R.D. Boutin, and T. Minas, Postoperative magnetic resonance imaging of articular cartilage repair. Semin Musculoskelet Radiol, 2001. 5(4): p. 345-63.*
89. *Domayer, S.E., G.H. Welsch, R. Dorotka, T.C. Mamisch, S. Marlovits, P. Szomolanyi, et al., MRI monitoring of cartilage repair in the knee: a review. Semin Musculoskelet Radiol, 2008. 12(4): p. 302-17.*
90. *Trattnig, S., V. Mlynarik, M. Huber, A. Ba-Ssalamah, S. Puig, and H. Imhof, Magnetic resonance imaging of articular cartilage and evaluation of cartilage disease. Invest Radiol, 2000. 35(10): p. 595-601.*
91. *Ramappa, A.J., T.J. Gill, C.H. Bradford, C.P. Ho, and J.R. Steadman, Magnetic resonance imaging to assess knee cartilage repair tissue after microfracture of chondral defects. J Knee Surg, 2007. 20(3): p. 228-34.*
92. *Link, T.M., C.A. Sell, J.N. Masi, C. Phan, D. Newitt, Y. Lu, et al., 3.0 vs 1.5 T MRI in the detection of focal cartilage pathology--ROC analysis in an experimental model. Osteoarthritis Cartilage, 2006. 14(1): p. 63-70.*
93. *Masi, J.N., C.A. Sell, C. Phan, E. Han, D. Newitt, L. Steinbach, et al., Cartilage MR imaging at 3.0 versus that at 1.5 T: preliminary results in a porcine model. Radiology, 2005. 236(1): p. 140-50.*
94. *Link, T.M., J. Mischung, K. Wortler, A. Burkart, E.J. Rummeny, and A.B. Imhoff, Normal and pathological MR findings in osteochondral autografts with longitudinal follow-up. Eur Radiol, 2006. 16(1): p. 88-96.*

95. Herber, S., M. Runkel, M.B. Pitton, P. Kalden, M. Thelen, and K.F. Kreitner, [Indirect MR-arthrography in the follow up of autologous osteochondral transplantation]. Rofo, 2003. 175(2): p. 226-33.
96. Sanders, T.G., K.D. Mentzer, M.D. Miller, W.B. Morrison, S.E. Campbell, and B.J. Penrod, Autogenous osteochondral "plug" transfer for the treatment of focal chondral defects: postoperative MR appearance with clinical correlation. Skeletal Radiol, 2001. 30(10): p. 570-8.
97. Trattnig, S., K. Pinker, C. Krestan, C. Plank, S. Millington, and S. Marlovits, Matrix-based autologous chondrocyte implantation for cartilage repair with HyalograftC: two-year follow-up by magnetic resonance imaging. Eur J Radiol, 2006. 57(1): p. 9-15.
98. Haddo, O., S. Mahroof, D. Higgs, L. David, J. Pringle, M. Bayliss, et al., The use of chondrogide membrane in autologous chondrocyte implantation. Knee, 2004. 11(1): p. 51-5.
99. Minas, T. and L. Peterson, Advanced techniques in autologous chondrocyte transplantation. Clin Sports Med, 1999. 18(1): p. 13-44, v-vi.
100. Minas, T. and R. Chiu, Autologous chondrocyte implantation. Am J Knee Surg, 2000. 13(1): p. 41-50.
101. Gold, G.E., A.G. Bergman, J.M. Pauly, P. Lang, R.K. Butts, C.F. Beaulieu, et al., Magnetic resonance imaging of knee cartilage repair. Top Magn Reson Imaging, 1998. 9(6): p. 377-92.
102. James, S.L., D.A. Connell, A. Saifuddin, J.A. Skinner, and T.W. Briggs, MR imaging of autologous chondrocyte implantation of the knee. Eur Radiol, 2006. 16(5): p. 1022-30.
103. Brown, W.E., H.G. Potter, R.G. Marx, T.L. Wickiewicz, and R.F. Warren, Magnetic resonance imaging appearance of cartilage repair in the knee. Clin Orthop Relat Res, 2004(422): p. 214-23.
104. Gold, G.E., B.A. Hargreaves, K.J. Stevens, and C.F. Beaulieu, Advanced magnetic resonance imaging of articular cartilage. Orthop Clin North Am, 2006. 37(3): p. 331-47, vi.
105. Schweitzer, M.E. and L.M. White, Does altered biomechanics cause marrow edema? Radiology, 1996. 198(3): p. 851-3.
106. Marlovits, S. and S. Trattnig, Cartilage repair. Eur J Radiol, 2006. 57(1): p. 1-2.
107. Marlovits, S., P. Singer, P. Zeller, I. Mandl, J. Haller, and S. Trattnig, Magnetic resonance observation of cartilage repair tissue (MOCART) for the evaluation of autologous chondrocyte transplantation: determination of interobserver variability and correlation to clinical outcome after 2 years. Eur J Radiol, 2006. 57(1): p. 16-23.
108. Trattnig, S., S.A. Millington, P. Szomolanyi, and S. Marlovits, MR imaging of osteochondral grafts and autologous chondrocyte implantation. Eur Radiol, 2007. 17(1): p. 103-18.
109. Trattnig, S., A. Ba-Ssalamah, K. Pinker, C. Plank, V. Vecsei, and S. Marlovits, Matrix-based autologous chondrocyte implantation for cartilage repair: noninvasive monitoring by high-resolution magnetic resonance imaging. Magn Reson Imaging, 2005. 23(7): p. 779-87.
110. Winalski, C.S. and K.B. Gupta, Magnetic resonance imaging of focal articular cartilage lesions. Top Magn Reson Imaging, 2003. 14(2): p. 131-44.
111. Glaser, C., T. Mendlik, J. Dinges, J. Weber, R. Stahl, C. Trumm, et al., Global and regional reproducibility of T2 relaxation time measurements in human patellar cartilage. Magn Reson Med, 2006. 56(3): p. 527-34.
112. Mosher, T.J. and B.J. Dardzinski, Cartilage MRI T2 relaxation time mapping: overview and applications. Semin Musculoskelet Radiol, 2004. 8(4): p. 355-68.
113. Lusse, S., H. Claassen, T. Gehrke, J. Hassenpflug, M. Schunke, M. Heller, et al., Evaluation of water content by spatially resolved transverse relaxation times of human articular cartilage. Magn Reson Imaging, 2000. 18(4): p. 423-30.
114. Menezes, N.M., M.L. Gray, J.R. Hartke, and D. Burstein, T2 and T1rho MRI in articular cartilage systems. Magn Reson Med, 2004. 51(3): p. 503-9.
115. Xia, Y., J.B. Moody, and H. Alhadlaq, Orientational dependence of T2 relaxation in articular cartilage: A microscopic MRI (microMRI) study. Magn Reson Med, 2002. 48(3): p. 460-9.

116. Dardzinski, B.J., T.J. Mosher, S. Li, M.A. Van Slyke, and M.B. Smith, Spatial variation of T2 in human articular cartilage. Radiology, 1997. 205(2): p. 546-50.
117. Watrin-Pinzano, A., J.P. Ruaud, Y. Cheli, P. Gonord, L. Grossin, I. Bettembourg-Brault, et al., Evaluation of cartilage repair tissue after biomaterial implantation in rat patella by using T2 mapping. Magma, 2004. 17(3-6): p. 219-28.
118. Goodwin, D.W., Y.Z. Wadghiri, and J.F. Dunn, Micro-imaging of articular cartilage: T2, proton density, and the magic angle effect. Acad Radiol, 1998. 5(11): p. 790-8.
119. Goodwin, D.W., H. Zhu, and J.F. Dunn, In vitro MR imaging of hyaline cartilage: correlation with scanning electron microscopy. AJR Am J Roentgenol, 2000. 174(2): p. 405-9.
120. Grunder, W., MRI assessment of cartilage ultrastructure. NMR Biomed, 2006. 19(7): p. 855-76.
121. Nissi, M.J., J. Rieppo, J. Toyras, M.S. Laasanen, I. Kiviranta, J.S. Jurvelin, et al., T(2) relaxation time mapping reveals age- and species-related diversity of collagen network architecture in articular cartilage. Osteoarthritis Cartilage, 2006. 14(12): p. 1265-71.
122. Shinar, H. and G. Navon, Multinuclear NMR and microscopic MRI studies of the articular cartilage nanostructure. NMR Biomed, 2006. 19(7): p. 877-93.
123. Goebel, J.C., A. Watrin-Pinzano, I. Bettembourg-Brault, F. Odille, J. Felblinger, I. Chary-Valckenaere, et al., Age-related quantitative MRI changes in healthy cartilage: preliminary results. Biorheology, 2006. 43(3-4): p. 547-51.
124. Mosher, T.J., B.J. Dardzinski, and M.B. Smith, Human articular cartilage: influence of aging and early symptomatic degeneration on the spatial variation of T2-- preliminary findings at 3 T. Radiology, 2000. 214(1): p. 259-66.
125. Mosher, T.J., Y. Liu, Q.X. Yang, J. Yao, R. Smith, B.J. Dardzinski, et al., Age dependency of cartilage magnetic resonance imaging T2 relaxation times in asymptomatic women. Arthritis Rheum, 2004. 50(9): p. 2820-8.
126. White, L.M., M.S. Sussman, M. Hurtig, L. Probyn, G. Tomlinson, and R. Kandel, Cartilage T2 assessment: differentiation of normal hyaline cartilage and reparative tissue after arthroscopic cartilage repair in equine subjects. Radiology, 2006. 241(2): p. 407-14.
127. Trattnig, S., T.C. Mamisch, G.H. Welsch, C. Glaser, P. Szomolanyi, S. Gebetsroither, et al., Quantitative T2 mapping of matrix-associated autologous chondrocyte transplantation at 3 Tesla: an in vivo cross-sectional study. Invest Radiol, 2007. 42(6): p. 442-8.
128. Kurkijarvi, J.E., L. Mattila, R.O. Ojala, A.I. Vasara, J.S. Jurvelin, I. Kiviranta, et al., Evaluation of cartilage repair in the distal femur after autologous chondrocyte transplantation using T2 relaxation time and dGEMRIC. Osteoarthritis Cartilage, 2007. 15(4): p. 372-8.
129. Maier, C.F., S.G. Tan, H. Hariharan, and H.G. Potter, T2 quantitation of articular cartilage at 1.5 T. J Magn Reson Imaging, 2003. 17(3): p. 358-64.
130. Pai, A., X. Li, and S. Majumdar, A comparative study at 3 T of sequence dependence of T2 quantitation in the knee. Magn Reson Imaging, 2008. 26(9): p. 1215-20.
131. Glaser, C., A. Horng, T. Mendlik, S. Weckbach, R.T. Hoffmann, S. Wagner, et al., [T2 relaxation time in patellar cartilage--global and regional reproducibility at 1.5 tesla and 3 tesla]. Rofo, 2007. 179(2): p. 146-52.
132. Kim, Y.J., D. Jaramillo, M.B. Millis, M.L. Gray, and D. Burstein, Assessment of early osteoarthritis in hip dysplasia with delayed gadolinium-enhanced magnetic resonance imaging of cartilage. J Bone Joint Surg Am, 2003. 85-A(10): p. 1987-92.
133. Tiderius, C.J., L.E. Olsson, P. Leander, O. Ekberg, and L. Dahlberg, Delayed gadolinium-enhanced MRI of cartilage (dGEMRIC) in early knee osteoarthritis. Magn Reson Med, 2003. 49(3): p. 488-92.
134. Roos, E.M. and L. Dahlberg, Positive effects of moderate exercise on glycosaminoglycan content in knee cartilage: a four-month, randomized, controlled trial in patients at risk of osteoarthritis. Arthritis Rheum, 2005. 52(11): p. 3507-14.
135. Cunningham, T., R. Jessel, D. Zurakowski, M.B. Millis, and Y.J. Kim, Delayed gadolinium-enhanced magnetic resonance imaging of cartilage to predict early failure of Bernese periacetabular osteotomy for hip dysplasia. J Bone Joint Surg Am, 2006. 88(7): p. 1540-8.

136. *McKenzie, C.A., A. Williams, P.V. Prasad, and D. Burstein, Three-dimensional delayed gadolinium-enhanced MRI of cartilage (dGEMRIC) at 1.5T and 3.0T. J Magn Reson Imaging, 2006. 24(4): p. 928-33.*
137. *Kimelman, T., A. Vu, P. Storey, C. McKenzie, D. Burstein, and P. Prasad, Three-dimensional T1 mapping for dGEMRIC at 3.0 T using the Look Locker method. Invest Radiol, 2006. 41(2): p. 198-203.*
138. *Watanabe, A., Y. Wada, T. Obata, T. Ueda, M. Tamura, H. Ikehira, et al., Delayed gadolinium-enhanced MR to determine glycosaminoglycan concentration in reparative cartilage after autologous chondrocyte implantation: preliminary results. Radiology, 2006. 239(1): p. 201-8.*
139. *Gillis, A., A. Bashir, B. McKeon, A. Scheller, M.L. Gray, and D. Burstein, Magnetic resonance imaging of relative glycosaminoglycan distribution in patients with autologous chondrocyte transplants. Invest Radiol, 2001. 36(12): p. 743-8.*
140. *Trattnig, S., S. Marlovits, S. Gebetsroither, P. Szomolanyi, G.H. Welsch, E. Salomonowitz, et al., Three-dimensional delayed gadolinium-enhanced MRI of cartilage (dGEMRIC) for in vivo evaluation of reparative cartilage after matrix-associated autologous chondrocyte transplantation at 3.0T: Preliminary results. J Magn Reson Imaging, 2007. 26(4): p. 974-82.*
141. *Mamisch, T.C., M. Dudda, T. Hughes, D. Burstein, and Y.J. Kim, Comparison of delayed gadolinium enhanced MRI of cartilage (dGEMRIC) using inversion recovery and fast T1 mapping sequences. Magn Reson Med, 2008. 60(4): p. 768-73.*
142. *Multanen, J., E. Rauvala, E. Lammentausta, R. Ojala, I. Kiviranta, A. Hakkinen, et al., Reproducibility of imaging human knee cartilage by delayed gadolinium-enhanced MRI of cartilage (dGEMRIC) at 1.5 Tesla. Osteoarthritis Cartilage, 2009. 17(5): p. 559-64.*
143. *Muhlenweg, M., G. Schaefers, and S. Trattnig, [Safety aspects in high-field magnetic resonance imaging]. Radiologe, 2008. 48(3): p. 258-67.*
144. *Michaely, H.J., H.S. Thomsen, M.F. Reiser, and S.O. Schoenberg, [Nephrogenic systemic fibrosis (NSF)--implications for radiology]. Radiologe, 2007. 47(9): p. 785-93.*
145. *Campoccia, D., P. Doherty, M. Radice, P. Brun, G. Abatangelo, and D.F. Williams, Semisynthetic resorbable materials from hyaluronan esterification. Biomaterials, 1998. 19(23): p. 2101-27.*
146. *Girotto, D., S. Urbani, P. Brun, D. Renier, R. Barbucci, and G. Abatangelo, Tissue-specific gene expression in chondrocytes grown on three-dimensional hyaluronic acid scaffolds. Biomaterials, 2003. 24(19): p. 3265-75.*
147. *Benedetti, L., R. Cortivo, T. Berti, A. Berti, F. Pea, M. Mazzo, et al., Biocompatibility and biodegradation of different hyaluronan derivatives (Hyaff) implanted in rats. Biomaterials, 1993. 14(15): p. 1154-60.*
148. *Eckstein, F., M. Kunz, M. Schutzer, M. Hudelmaier, R.D. Jackson, J. Yu, et al., Two year longitudinal change and test-retest-precision of knee cartilage morphology in a pilot study for the osteoarthritis initiative. Osteoarthritis Cartilage, 2007. 15(11): p. 1326-32.*
149. *Gambarota, G., B.E. Cairns, C.B. Berde, and R.V. Mulkern, Osmotic effects on the T2 relaxation decay of in vivo muscle. Magn Reson Med, 2001. 46(3): p. 592-9.*
150. *Jones, C.K., Q.S. Xiang, K.P. Whittall, and A.L. MacKay, Linear combination of multiecho data: short T2 component selection. Magn Reson Med, 2004. 51(3): p. 495-502.*
151. *Lysholm, J. and J. Gillquist, Evaluation of knee ligament surgery results with special emphasis on use of a scoring scale. Am J Sports Med, 1982. 10(3): p. 150-4.*
152. *Kocher, M.S., J.R. Steadman, K.K. Briggs, W.I. Sterett, and R.J. Hawkins, Reliability, validity, and responsiveness of the Lysholm knee scale for various chondral disorders of the knee. J Bone Joint Surg Am, 2004. 86-A(6): p. 1139-45.*
153. *Briggs, K.K., M.S. Kocher, W.G. Rodkey, and J.R. Steadman, Reliability, validity, and responsiveness of the Lysholm knee score and Tegner activity scale for patients with meniscal injury of the knee. J Bone Joint Surg Am, 2006. 88(4): p. 698-705.*
154. *Hefti, F., W. Muller, R.P. Jakob, and H.U. Staubli, Evaluation of knee ligament injuries with the IKDC form. Knee Surg Sports Traumatol Arthrosc, 1993. 1(3-4): p. 226-34.*

155. Roos, E., Rigorous statistical reliability, validity, and responsiveness testing of the Cincinnati Knee Rating System in 350 subjects with uninjured, injured, or anterior cruciate ligament-reconstructed knee. Am J Sports Med, 2000. 28(3): p. 436-8.
156. Higgins, L.D., M.K. Taylor, D. Park, N. Ghodadra, M. Marchant, R. Pietrobon, et al., Reliability and validity of the International Knee Documentation Committee (IKDC) Subjective Knee Form. Joint Bone Spine, 2007. 74(6): p. 594-9.
157. Anderson, A.F., J.J. Irrgang, M.S. Kocher, B.J. Mann, and J.J. Harrast, The International Knee Documentation Committee Subjective Knee Evaluation Form: normative data. Am J Sports Med, 2006. 34(1): p. 128-35.
158. Irrgang, J.J., A.F. Anderson, A.L. Boland, C.D. Harner, M. Kurosaka, P. Neyret, et al., Development and validation of the international knee documentation committee subjective knee form. Am J Sports Med, 2001. 29(5): p. 600-13.
159. Williams A, M.B., Krishnan N, Gray M, McKenzie C, Burstein D, Suitability of T1Gd as the "dGEMRIC Index" at 1.5 and 3.0T. Proc Int Soc Magn Reson Med ; 2619 2007.
160. Domayer, S.E., G.H. Welsch, S. Nehrer, C. Chiari, R. Dorotka, P. Szomolanyi, et al., T2 mapping and dGEMRIC after autologous chondrocyte implantation with a fibrin-based scaffold in the knee: Preliminary results. Eur J Radiol, 2009.
161. Welsch, G.H., T.C. Mamisch, S.E. Domayer, R. Dorotka, F. Kutscha-Lissberg, S. Marlovits, et al., Cartilage T2 assessment at 3-T MR imaging: in vivo differentiation of normal hyaline cartilage from reparative tissue after two cartilage repair procedures--initial experience. Radiology, 2008. 247(1): p. 154-61.
162. Trattnig, S., T.C. Mamisch, K. Pinker, S. Domayer, P. Szomolanyi, S. Marlovits, et al., Differentiating normal hyaline cartilage from post-surgical repair tissue using fast gradient echo imaging in delayed gadolinium-enhanced MRI (dGEMRIC) at 3 Tesla. Eur Radiol, 2008. 18(6): p. 1251-9.
163. Domayer, S.E., F. Kutscha-Lissberg, G. Welsch, R. Dorotka, S. Nehrer, C. Gabler, et al., T2 mapping in the knee after microfracture at 3.0 T: correlation of global T2 values and clinical outcome - preliminary results. Osteoarthritis Cartilage, 2008. 16(8): p. 903-8.
164. Takao, M., M. Ochi, K. Naito, Y. Uchio, T. Kono, and K. Oae, Arthroscopic drilling for chondral, subchondral, and combined chondral-subchondral lesions of the talar dome. Arthroscopy, 2003. 19(5): p. 524-30.
165. Sun, P.Z., T. Benner, A. Kumar, and A.G. Sorensen, Investigation of optimizing and translating pH-sensitive pulsed-chemical exchange saturation transfer (CEST) imaging to a 3T clinical scanner. Magn Reson Med, 2008. 60(4): p. 834-41.
166. Sun, P.Z. and A.G. Sorensen, Imaging pH using the chemical exchange saturation transfer (CEST) MRI: Correction of concomitant RF irradiation effects to quantify CEST MRI for chemical exchange rate and pH. Magn Reson Med, 2008. 60(2): p. 390-7.
167. Zhang, S., X. Zhu, Z. Chen, C. Cai, T. Lin, and J. Zhong, Improvement in the contrast of CEST MRI via intermolecular double quantum coherences. Phys Med Biol, 2008. 53(14): p. N287-96.
168. Mamisch, T.C., M.I. Menzel, G.H. Welsch, B. Bittersohl, E. Salomonowitz, P. Szomolanyi, et al., Steady-state diffusion imaging for MR in-vivo evaluation of reparative cartilage after matrix-associated autologous chondrocyte transplantation at 3 tesla-Preliminary results. Eur J Radiol, 2008. 65(1): p. 72-9.
169. Grigolo, B., L. Roseti, M. Fiorini, M. Fini, G. Giavaresi, N.N. Aldini, et al., Transplantation of chondrocytes seeded on a hyaluronan derivative (hyaff-11) into cartilage defects in rabbits. Biomaterials, 2001. 22(17): p. 2417-24.
170. Solchaga, L.A., J.E. Dennis, V.M. Goldberg, and A.I. Caplan, Hyaluronic acid-based polymers as cell carriers for tissue-engineered repair of bone and cartilage. J Orthop Res, 1999. 17(2): p. 205-13.
171. Manfredini, M., F. Zerbinati, A. Gildone, and R. Faccini, Autologous chondrocyte implantation: a comparison between an open periosteal-covered and an arthroscopic matrix-guided technique. Acta Orthop Belg, 2007. 73(2): p. 207-18.
172. Nehrer, S., C. Chiari, S. Domayer, H. Barkay, and A. Yayon, Results of chondrocyte implantation with a fibrin-hyaluronan matrix: a preliminary study. Clin Orthop Relat Res, 2008. 466(8): p. 1849-55.

173. *Trattnig S, M.T., Pinker K, Domayer S, Szomolanyi P, Marlovits S, Kutscha-Lissberg F, Welsch GH, Differentiating normal hyaline cartilage from post-surgical repair tissue using fast gradient echo imaging in delayed gadolinium enhanced MRI - (dGEMRIC) at 3 Tesla. Eur Radiol, 2008. in press.*
174. *Smith, H.E., T.J. Mosher, B.J. Dardzinski, B.G. Collins, C.M. Collins, Q.X. Yang, et al., Spatial variation in cartilage T2 of the knee. J Magn Reson Imaging, 2001. 14(1): p. 50-5.*
175. *Xia, Y., J.B. Moody, N. Burton-Wurster, and G. Lust, Quantitative in situ correlation between microscopic MRI and polarized light microscopy studies of articular cartilage. Osteoarthritis Cartilage, 2001. 9(5): p. 393-406.*
176. *Kim, Y.J., S. Bixby, T.C. Mamisch, J.C. Clohisy, and J.C. Carlisle, Imaging structural abnormalities in the hip joint: instability and impingement as a cause of osteoarthritis. Semin Musculoskelet Radiol, 2008. 12(4): p. 334-45.*
177. *Williams, A., S.K. Shetty, D. Burstein, C.S. Day, and C. McKenzie, Delayed gadolinium enhanced MRI of cartilage (dGEMRIC) of the first carpometacarpal (1CMC) joint: a feasibility study. Osteoarthritis Cartilage, 2008. 16(4): p. 530-2.*
178. *Welsch, G.H., T.C. Mamisch, T. Hughes, C. Zilkens, S. Quirbach, K. Scheffler, et al., In vivo biochemical 7.0 Tesla magnetic resonance: preliminary results of dGEMRIC, zonal T2, and T2* mapping of articular cartilage. Invest Radiol, 2008. 43(9): p. 619-26.*
179. *Mithoefer, K., R.J. Williams, 3rd, R.F. Warren, H.G. Potter, C.R. Spock, E.C. Jones, et al., Chondral resurfacing of articular cartilage defects in the knee with the microfracture technique. Surgical technique. J Bone Joint Surg Am, 2006. 88 Suppl 1 Pt 2: p. 294-304.*

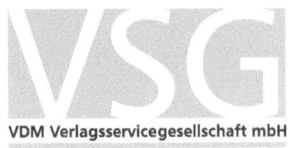

Die VDM Verlagsservicegesellschaft sucht für wissenschaftliche Verlage abgeschlossene und herausragende

Dissertationen, Habilitationen, Diplomarbeiten, Master Theses, Magisterarbeiten usw.

für die kostenlose Publikation als Fachbuch.

Sie verfügen über eine Arbeit, die hohen inhaltlichen und formalen Ansprüchen genügt, und haben Interesse an einer honorarvergüteten Publikation?

Dann senden Sie bitte erste Informationen über sich und Ihre Arbeit per Email an *info@vdm-vsg.de*.

Sie erhalten kurzfristig unser Feedback!

VDM Verlagsservicegesellschaft mbH
Dudweiler Landstr. 99   Telefon +49 681 3720 174
D - 66123 Saarbrücken   Fax   +49 681 3720 1749
www.vdm-vsg.de

Die VDM Verlagsservicegesellschaft mbH vertritt

 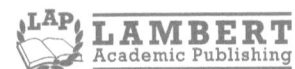 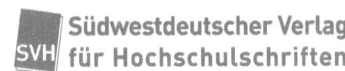

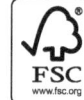
MIX
Papier aus verantwortungsvollen Quellen
Paper from responsible sources
FSC® C105338

Printed by Books on Demand GmbH, Norderstedt / Germany